WP555

# THERAPEUTIC
# HYSTEROSCOPY
Indications and Techniques

# THERAPEUTIC HYSTEROSCOPY
## Indications and Techniques

**ALVIN M. SIEGLER, M.D., D.Sc.**
Clinical Professor
Department of Obstetrics and Gynecology
State University of New York
Health Science Center at Brooklyn
Brooklyn, New York

**RAFAEL F. VALLE, M.D.**
Associate Professor
Department of Obstetrics and Gynecology
Northwestern University Medical School
Chicago, Illinois

**HANS J. LINDEMANN, M.D.**
Professor
Department of Obstetrics and Gynecology
University of Hamburg
Hamburg, West Germany

**LUCA MENCAGLIA, M.D.**
Assistant Professor
Department of Obstetrics and Gynecology
University of Perugia
Florence, Italy

*With 231 illustrations*

## THE C. V. MOSBY COMPANY

St. Louis • Baltimore • Philadelphia • Toronto    1990

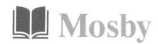 Mosby

*Editor* Stephanie Bircher Manning
*Assistant Editor* Anne Gunter
*Project Manager* Carol Sullivan Wiseman
*Senior Production Editor* Barbara Bowes Merritt
*Designer* Candace Conner

Printed in the United States of America

The C. V. Mosby Company
11830 Westline Industrial Drive, St. Louis, Missouri 63146

**Library of Congress Cataloging-in-Publication Data**

Therapeutic hysteroscopy : indications and techniques / editor, Alvin M. Siegler ; associate editors, Rafael F. Valle, Hans J. Lindemann, Luca Mencaglia.

   p.  cm.
Includes bibliographical references.
ISBN 0-8016-5504-8

   1.  Hysteroscopy.  I.  Siegler, Alvin M. (Alvin Morton).
[DNLM: 1.  Endoscopy—instrumentation.  2.  Endoscopy—methods.
3.  Uterine Diseases—diagnosis.  4.  Uterine Diseases—therapy.
WP 400 061]
RG304.5.H97064   1990
618.1′45—dc20
DNLM/DLC
for Library of Congress
                                        89-13339
                                           CIP

VT/W/W  9  8  7  6  5  4  3  2  1

# *Foreword*

Amazing advancements in the technology of pelvic endoscopy have occurred over the past 2 decades. Today's gynecologists accurately diagnose and treat many pelvic disorders by means of laparoscopy, culdoscopy, salpingoscopy, and hysteroscopy. For many years hysteroscopy was hindered by limitations. The problems of inadequate lighting and insufficient uterine distention have been overcome, and today this form of endoscopy has gained widespread acceptance. The increasing popularity of this instrumentation has created a demand for a definitive textbook on the principles of diagnostic and therapeutic hysteroscopy.

The significant contributions of Alvin M. Siegler, Rafael F. Valle, Hans J. Lindemann, and Luca Mencaglia to the advancements in laparoscopy and hysteroscopy have established them as international authorities on endoscopy. They helped pioneer the use of hysteroscopy and today are much sought after lecturers and medical writers. They are superbly qualified to write a state-of-the-art textbook on this type of endoscopy and have developed a well-written, smooth-flowing textbook.

The initial chapters describe the latest advancements in instrumentation and the refinements in media distention. Each succeeding, well-referenced chapter deals with specific disorders that lend themselves to management by hysteroscopy, such as metroplasty, intrauterine adhesions, and abnormal uterine bleeding. The many excellent illustrations fully complement the text and make it enjoyable to read. It represents a current, comprehensive source of ready information on hysteroscopy.

This important book is designed for serious students of reproductive surgery and all those interested in reproductive medicine. It will be a welcome addition to the personal libraries of residents-in-training, clinicians, and educators.

Roger D. Kempers, M.D.
Professor of Obstetrics and Gynecology
Mayo Medical School
Consultant, Department of Obstetrics and Gynecology
Mayo Clinic
Rochester, Minnesota

# Preface

Hysteroscopy has evolved from a diagnostic procedure into a therapeutic approach for a variety of gynecologic conditions. Instruments specifically designed for hysteroscopic operative procedures have been developed. The indications for therapeutic hysteroscopy are increasing and its proper applications can improve the patient's gynecologic care. These facts should stimulate the gynecologist to become proficient with hysteroscopy for the diagnosis and the treatment of many intrauterine abnormalities.

There are major advantages to a transcervical approach including the avoidance of a laparotomy with the potential sequelae that can follow an abdominal operation. Hysteroscopic operative techniques have been refined, and, with experience, good postoperative results and low morbidity have become evident.

A hysteroscopic metroplasty can be performed on the septate uterus to facilitate and improve the subsequent reproductive outcome. In selected patients, symptomatic, submucous, nonmalignant tumors can be located and removed under hysteroscopic control. The accepted method of therapy for intrauterine adhesions requires their identification and subsequent lysis using the hysteroscope and accessory instruments. Foreign bodies "lost" in the uterine cavity and occult or embedded IUDs can be identified and removed with minimal trauma under direct vision. Endometrial ablation is a procedure used to induce amenorrhea or hypomenorrhea in patients experiencing abnormal uterine bleeding, who are not candidates for a hysterectomy, and have not responded to medical therapy or curettage. This operation can be accomplished using either electrosurgery or laser photocoagulation.

As the physician's approach to some of these intrauterine problems is refined and the technique becomes more widespread, other therapeutic applications of the hysteroscope are being investigated. These include tubal cannulation and the application of new reproductive technology such as placement of gametes into the fallopian tubes and embryo transfer. Because of the simplicity of a transcervical approach to the uterotubal ostia, hysteroscopy has been utilized as a possible method for sterilization or a technique for contraception.

Each of these procedures is fully described in this book, and the trained hysteroscopist should be able to gradually incorporate some of them into the practice of gynecologic endoscopy.

We emphasize that the gynecologist must have previously become proficient using hysteroscopy as a diagnostic method before undertaking operative, therapeutic techniques. The time has come for the use of the hysteroscope to be expanded to treat many gynecologic diseases that heretofore required a laparotomy, which involves longer hospitalization, increased costs, and the possible postoperative formation of pelvic adhesions.

Alvin M. Siegler
Rafael F. Valle
Hans J. Lindemann
Luca Mencaglia

# Acknowledgments

The concept, development, and publication of this book required the efforts and cooperation of many colleagues and friends. We wish to express our gratitude to those physicians who graciously permitted us to use some of their illustrations so our book could be as complete as possible.

A special thanks is given to Leon Chesley, Ph.D., in appreciation for his willingness to read the entire manuscript and improve our ability to express ourselves in a more concise manner.

The Department of Medical Illustrations of the State University of New York, Health Science Center at Brooklyn was most diligent in their efforts to reproduce and insure the quality of the illustrations.

We wish to acknowledge with appreciation the efforts of Stephanie Manning of The C.V. Mosby Company who inspired us to write this book and facilitated its publication. Barbara Merritt, Senior Production Editor, collated the text and illustrations with patience and a dedication to excellence.

Finally we express an everlasting thanks to our families, to Marcia, Hertha, and Laura who always have encouraged efforts to improve the quality of health care for women.

# Contents

# 1 Historical Survey

Describing himself as a Doctor of Medicine and Surgery, a member of various learned societies, a practicing physician and obstetrician from Frankfurt-am-Main, Bozzini[5] published a classical treatise in 1807 on the "light conductor." In the preface he wrote "every invention owes its origin to a happy combination of various circumstances; it is always born like a child, and like a child it keeps becoming more nearly perfect by stepwise progression." The light-conductor was a vase-shaped lantern made of tin and covered with leather (Fig. 1-1). In the center of the lantern was a wax candle fixed in a metal tube that was forced upward by a spring. The lantern had three apertures: two on one side separated by a septum and one on the opposite side.

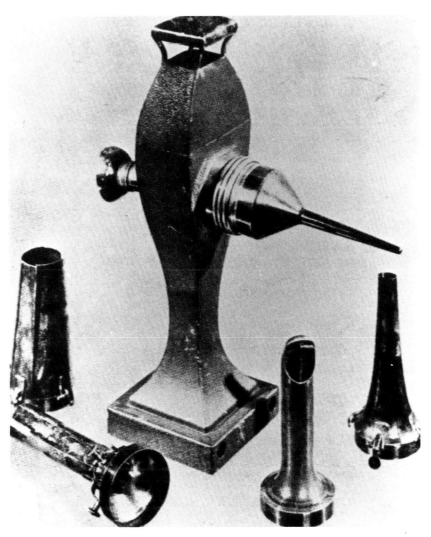

*FIG. 1-1* Instruments described by Bozzini in 1807 treatise.[5] Vase-shaped apparatus was 37 cm high, 3.2 cm in depth, and 8 cm in width.

The flame from the candle was at the left, below the two apertures that served as an outlet for the different specula. The specula were also divided by a septum; one canal conducted the light into the hollow organs, the other one made observation possible. Bozzini described this apparatus as "a simple device for the illumination of inner cavities and interstices of the living animal body." He declared that surgical diagnoses would become more certain, since the extent, the character, and the form of tumors and diseased states could be seen. "The trained touch of the obstetrician, now reinforced by the eye or guided by it, will scarcely be capable of a mistake any longer. Uterine hemorrhages which develop from various spots in the uterus, their site of origin and extent can be determined and more effective measures applied." Successful experiments were done on patients who had diseases of the rectum and uterus but Bozzini's invention fell victim to professional jealousy, court intrigue, and the battle between conservatism and liberalism in the medical community. Bozzini's early death at 35 years of age from typhoid fever ended his attempts to improve and fight for the light conductor, but his idea of endoscopy survived him (Fig. 1-2).[33]

Aubinais[2] was apparently the first person to describe an attempt to look inside the uterus of a pregnant woman. In 1863, using candle light reflected by a mirror, he was able to look through the anterior abdominal wall. He termed the procedure *uteroscopy*. Two years later Désormeaux,[8] using an endoscope, reported on the diagnosis and treatment of diseases of the urethra and bladder. A cylindrical tube was inserted into the urinary bladder and a mirror was used to reflect light.

In 1869, Pantaleoni performed an endoscopic examination of the uterine cavity in a 60-year-old patient who complained of postmenopausal bleeding.[30] Preoperatively he inserted a "sponge tent" to dilate the endocervical canal. Pantaleoni discovered "a polypous vegetation at the bottom of the cavity towards the posterior part of the fundus uteri." He used a slight variation of the cylindrical tube of Désormeaux that was 20 cm long and 12 mm wide. He then introduced a caustic substance through the tube. He believed that this technique brought a new system of exploration and cure.

No new advocates of this technique were forthcoming and 10 years later Munde,[27] professor of gynecology at Dartmouth College, wrote in his textbook, *Minor Surgical Gynecology*, that "if one compares the information derived from this way compared with that obtained by using the tip of the index finger, the proverbial eye of the gynecologist, then it has to be said that this fleeting glimpse is of little value." Munde used an instrument similar to the one devised by Skene for examining the urinary bladder.

Another 10 years passed before Morris[26] published a paper in *Transactions of the American Association of Obstetricians and Gynecologists* on the use of endoscopic tubes for inspection of the urinary bladder and the uterine cavity. He used a straight cylindrical tube of thin, silver-plated brass 22 cm long and 9 mm wide. The tube was beveled smoothly at the uterine (distal) end. The obturator inside the tube was withdrawn after the instrument had been introduced into the uterine cavity, leaving the hollow tube as the endoscope (Fig. 1-3). Morris observed the endometrium and the tubal ostia using a light reflected through an ordinary head mirror. Ancillary instruments could be used to remove pathologic specimens through the endoscope.

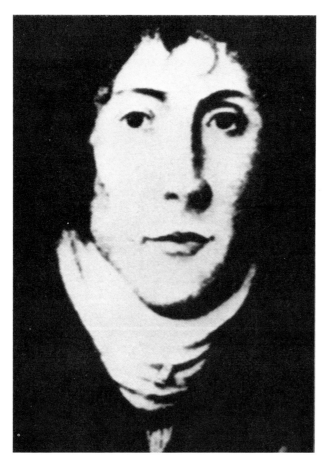

*FIG. 1-2* Self-portrait of Bozzini (about 1805) from the town archives in Frankfurt.[33] (From Rathert P, Lutzeyer W, and Goddwin WE: Philipp Bozzini (1773-1809) and the Lichtleiter, Urology 3:113, 1974.)

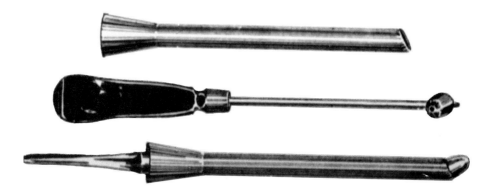

*FIG. 1-3* Instruments used by Morris in 1893 to perform hysteroscopy.[26]

Before the turn of the century, the first book on hysteroscopy was written by Duplay and Clado[9] (Fig. 1-4). This book with 28 illustrations described instruments, techniques, and clinical studies of 28 women. Duplay and Clado used an open-ended tube with a battery light source. Ten years later, another French physician, David,[7] wrote his master's thesis on hysteroscopy. For the first time a lens was built into the endoscope, but the illumination system was mounted externally. David explored the entire uterine cavity in a methodical fashion (Fig. 1-5). His thesis included color illustrations of abnormalities, intrauterine adhesions, polyps, submucous myomas, and even the appearance of a uterine perforation.

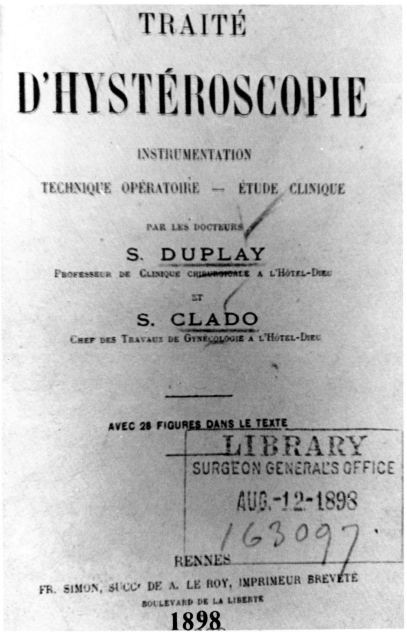

FIG. 1-4 Title page from original book written by Duplay and Clado in 1898.[9]

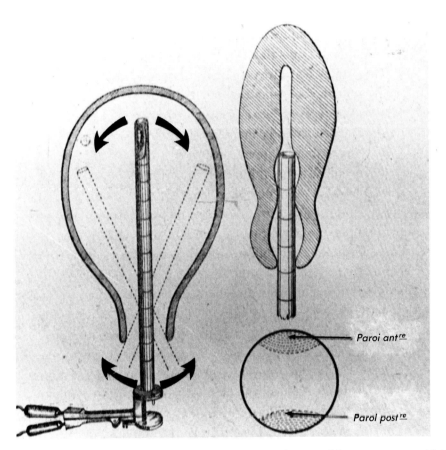

*FIG. 1-5* Schematic representation of manipulation of hysteroscope within the uterine cavity. (From David C: L'endoscopie utérine [hystéroscopie]. Applications au diagnostic et au traitement des affections intra-utérines. Master's thesis, University of Paris, Paris, 1908, G Jacques.)

During the next decade a light source became part of the endoscope. A water rinsing system was incorporated to distend the uterine cavity and to wash away the blood and mucus.[4] In 1925, Rubin[34] used carbon dioxide ($CO_2$) to distend the uterine cavities of 35 women in an office setting as part of individual infertility studies. He noted that $CO_2$ insufflation through a 15 Fr modified McCarthy cystourethroscope required an intrauterine pressure of about 60 mm Hg to distend the uterine cavity in a procedure lasting only a few minutes. Rubin described the potential values of endometroscopy for the following: (1) catheterization of the tubal ostia, (2) tubal cannulation to overcome proximal tubal obstruction, (3) cauterization as a method of tubal sterilization, and (4) the possible removal of submucous tumors.

Rubin's paper, presented before the fiftieth annual meeting of the American Gynecological Society in 1925, was discussed by Heineberg and Ansbach from Philadelphia, both of whom had used hysteroscopy in their practices for 10 years. Dickinson, the final discussant commented, "finally we can see the inside of the uterine cavity and the tubal ostia. Therefore this marks a tremendous advance."

Adequate illumination and sustained distention of the uterine cavity were problems that prevented consistent success with hysteroscopy. Except for the contributions by Heineberg,[17] Rubin,[34] and Norment,[28] the American literature contains meager information about hysteroscopy before 1950. The discovery of the cold quartz light source by Forestier et al.[13] in 1952 and fiberoptics by Hopkins and Kapany[18] in 1965 brought endoscopy to a new level of reproducibility (Table 1-1). The use of colloid media[23] and the re-introduction of $CO_2$ with a properly calibrated apparatus to control intra-uterine pressure and limit the flow rates to less than 100 ml/min improved the quality of the view of the uterine cavity and the safety of the procedure (Table 1-2).[19,31]

## FUTURE OF HYSTEROSCOPY

In the future, gynecologists must become convinced that hysteroscopy is valuable enough to be incorporated into clinical practice. For too many years and perhaps with good reason, there has been a reluctance to add this relatively minor, surgical procedure to the standard skills of the gynecologist. Having accomplished the diagnostic technique, the physician can proceed to develop skills of therapeutic hysteroscopy, including lysis of intrauterine adhesions, metroplasty, submucous myomectomy and polypectomy, and endometrial obliteration as therapy for menorrhagia. Therapeutic hysteroscopy has had a prolonged gestation. Perhaps the time has come to increase the use of this endoscopic method in selected patients to obviate the need for laparotomy, uterine incisions, and even hysterectomy.

*Table 1-1* One Hundred and Sixty Years in the Development of Hysteroscopy (1809-1969)

| Before 1900 | 1900-1909 | 1910-1919 | 1920-1929 |
|---|---|---|---|
| Aubinais[2] | David[7] | Heineberg[17] | Gauss[14] |
| Beuttner[4] | | Seymour[39] | Mickulicz-Radecki[24] |
| Bozzini[5] | | | Rubin[34] |
| Désormeaux[8] | | | Schroeder[37] |
| Duplay/Clado[9] | | | |
| Morris[26] | | | |
| Pantaleoni[30] | | | |

| 1930-1939 | 1940-1949 | 1950-1959 | 1960-1969 |
|---|---|---|---|
| Haselhorst[16] | Norment[28] | Bank[3] | Aguero[1] |
| Litwak[20] | | Englund[11] | Burnett[6] |
| Schack[35] | | Gribb[15] | Edström/Fernström[10] |
| Segond[38] | | Forestier[13] | Esposito[12] |
| | | Palmer[29] | Lyon[21] |
| | | Wulfson[41] | Marleschki[22] |
| | | | Mohri et al.[25] |
| | | | Schmidt-Matthiesen[36] |
| | | | Menken[23] |
| | | | Silander[40] |

*Table 1-2* Historical Development of Media for Hysteroscopy

| Author | Year | Contribution |
|---|---|---|
| Heineberg[17] | 1914 | Water rinsing system |
| Rubin[34] | 1925 | Insufflation with $CO_2$ |
| Gauss[14] | 1928 | Pressurized water rinsing system |
| Norment[28] | 1950 | Transparent plastic/rubber balloons |
| Marleschki[22] | 1966 | Glass shield (contact) |
| Menken[23] | 1968 | Polyvinylpyrrolidine |
| Edström/Fernström[10] | 1970 | High molecular dextran (Hyskon) |
| Lindemann[19] | 1971 | Pneumohysteroscopy with $CO_2$ |
| Porto/Gaujoux[31] | 1972 | Cervical adaptor with $CO_2$ |
| Quinones[32] | 1972 | 5% glucose solution |

*References*

1. Aguero O, Aure M, and Lopez R: Hysteroscopy in pregnant patient—a new diagnostic tool, Am J Obstet Gynecol 94:925, 1966.
2. Aubinais EJ: De l'uteroscopie, J Sect Med Soc Acad Loire Infer 39:71, 1863.
3. Bank EB: Erfahrungen mit der Metroskopie, Zentralb Gynäkol 82:866, 1960.
4. Beuttner O: Über Hysteroskopie, Zentralb Gynäkol 22:580, 1898.
5. Bozzini P: Der Lichtleiter oder Beschreibung einer einfachen Vorrichtung und ihrer Anwendung Erleuchtung innerer Höhlen und Zwischenräume des lebenden animalischen Körpers, Weimar, 1807, Landes-Industrie-Comptoir.
6. Burnett JE Jr: Hysteroscopy-controlled curettage for endometrial polyps, Obstet Gynecol 24:621, 1964.
7. David C: L'endoscopie utérine (hystéroscopie). Applications au diagnostic et au traitement des affections intra-uterines, master's thesis, University of Paris, Paris, 1908, G Jacques.
8. Désormeaux AJ: De l'endoscope et de ses applications au diagnostic et au traitement des affections de l'urètre et la vessie, Paris, 1865, Baillaire.
9. Duplay S and Clado S: Traite d'hystéroscopie, instrumentation, technique, operatoire, étude clinique, Rennes, 1898, Simon.
10. Edström K and Fernström I: The diagnostic possibilities of a modified hysteroscopic technique, Acta Obstet Gynecol Scand 49:327, 1970.
11. Englund S, Ingleman-Sundberg A, and Westin B: Hysteroscopy in diagnosis and treatment of bleeding, Gynecologia 143:217, 1957.
12. Esposito A: Une exploration gynécologique negligée: l'hystéroscopie, Gynecol Pract 19:167, 1968.
13. Forestier M, Gladu A, and Vulmiere J: Perfectionnements de l'endoscope médicale, Presse Med 60:1292, 1952.
14. Gauss GJ: Hysteroskopie, Arch Gynäkol 133:18, 1928.
15. Gribb JJ: Hysteroscopy: an aid in gynecologic diagnosis, Obstet Gynecol 15:593, 1960.
16. Haselhorst G: Unsere Erfahrungen mit der Hysteroskopie, Zentralb Gynäkol 59:2442, 1935.
17. Heineberg A: Uterine-endoscopy, an aid to precision in the diagnosis of intra-uterine disease, Surg Gynecol Obstet 18:513, 1914.
18. Hopkins HH and Kapany NS: Flexible fiberscope, using static scanning, Nature 173:39, 1954.
19. Lindemann HJ: Eine neue Untersuchungsmethode für die Hysteroskopie, Endoscopy 4:194, 1971.
20. Litwak B and Wiktorowskaja E: Regeneration der Uterusschleimhaut nach künstlichem Abort und hysteroskopisches Studium derselben, Monatschr Geburtsh Gynäkol 101:55, 1935.
21. Lyon FA: Intrauterine visualization by means of a hysteroscope, Am J Obstet Gynecol 90:443, 1964.
22. Marleschki V: Die moderne Zervikoskopie und Hysteroskopie, Zlb Gynäkol 88:637, 1966.
23. Menken FC: Fortschritte der gynäkologischen Endoskopie. In Demling L and Ottenjann R, eds: Fortschritte der Endoskopie, Stuttgart, 1969, FK Schattauer.
24. Mikulicz-Radecki F and Freund A: Ein neues Hysteroskop und seine praktische Anwendung in der Gynäkologie, Geburtsh Gynäkol 92:13, 1927.
25. Mohri T, Mohri C, and Yamadori F: The original production of the glass-fibre hysteroscope and a study of the intrauterine observation of the human fetus, things attached to the fetus and inner side of the uterus wall in late pregnancy and the beginning of delivery by means of hysteroscopy and its recording on film, J Jpn Obstet Gynecol Soc 15:76, 1968.
26. Morris RT: Endoscopic tubes for direct inspection of the bladder and uterus, Trans Am Assoc Obstet Gynecol 6:275, 1893.
27. Munde PF: Minor Surgical Gynecology, New York, 1880, W. Wood.
28. Norment WB: A study of the uterine cavity by direct observation and the uterogram, Am J Surg 60:56, 1943.
29. Palmer R: Un nouvel hystéroscope, Bull Fe Soc Gynecol Obstet Franc 9:300, 1957.

30. Pantaleoni DC: On endoscopic examination of the cavity of the womb, Med Press Circ 8:26, 1869.
31. Porto R and Gaujoux J: Une nouvelle méthode d'hystéroscopie: Instrumentation et technique, J Gynecol Obstet Biol Reprod 1:691, 1972.
32. Quinones RG, Alvarado-Diran A, and Aznar-Ramos R: Tubal catheterization: applications of a new technique, Am J Obstet Gynecol 114:674, 1972.
33. Rathert P, Lutzeyer W, and Goddwin WE: Philipp Bozzini (1773-1809) and the Lichtleiter, Urology 3:113, 1974.
34. Rubin IC: Uterine endoscopy, endometroscopy with the aid of uterine insufflation, Am J Obstet Gynecol 10:313, 1925.
35. Schack L: Unsere Erfahrungen mit der Hysteroskopie, Zentralb Gynäkol 60: 1810, 1936.
36. Schmidt-Matthiesen H: Die Hysteroskopie als klinische Routine Methode, Geburtsh Frauenhkd 26: 1498, 1966.
37. Schroeder C: Über den Aufbau und die Leistungen der Hysteroskopie, Arch Gynäkol 156:407, 1934.
38. Segond R: Hystéroscopie, Bull Soc Obstet Gynecol 23:709, 1934.
39. Seymour HF: Endoscopy of the uterus with a description of a hysteroscope, J Obstet Gynaecol Brit Emp 33:52, 1926.
40. Silander T: Hysteroscopy through a transparent rubber balloon, Surg Gynecol Obstet 114:125, 1962.
41. Wulfson NL: A hysteroscope, J Obstet Gynaecol Brit Emp 65:657, 1958.

# 2 *Instruments*

Hysteroscopy requires appropriate equipment, including an endoscope, a distending medium for panoramic hysteroscopy, an appropriate light source, and ancillary instruments for operative interventions.

## HYSTEROSCOPES

All hysteroscopes should enable the gynecologist to have an undistorted clear observation of the uterine cavity. They transmit light for illumination and carry the image to the viewer's eye. The optical components of the hysteroscope include lenses and prisms. The illumination component is provided by fiberoptics.[6,15,16] Until 1975 doublet and single lenses were used in some rigid hysteroscopes (Fig. 2-1). With the rod lens system designed by Hopkins,[9,10] the lens thickness is larger than its diameter with small air spaces in between (Fig. 2-2). This innovation provides a larger viewing angle. A brighter image is transmitted by the long cylinders of superior optical quality glass. Another system used is the graded refractory index (GRIN) system which includes a narrow rod of glass with a refractory index that progressively decreases from the axis to the periphery. The GRIN system is used predominately with slender optical systems such as needle endoscopes.[14]

The proximal end of the hysteroscope contains several important optical components. The prism is used to form an upright image of the object and the lens magnifies the image. The overall magnification of the endoscope is the product of the magnification of the objective lens and the eyepiece. Normal overall magnification of the panoramic hysteroscope is about unity at a normal working distance (about 200 mm). The magnification is inversely proportional to the distance of the object to the lens. The precise magnification for the hysteroscope can be determined only if the distance to the object is known and these objects (i.e., polyps, myomas, etc.) are located at different distances from the objective lens. Most rigid hysteroscopes generally do not employ variable focus optics, and the viewer must be capable of seeing large depth of field (images falling within the range of the accommodation of the eye between infinity and 250 mm). In addition, hysteroscopes are monocular, providing little depth perception for the viewer; interpretation of depth comes with experience.

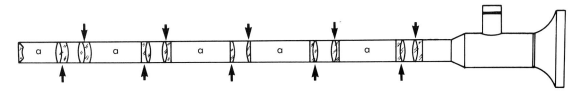

FIG. 2-1 Traditional "bead" optical system. *a*, Air, *arrows*, lens.

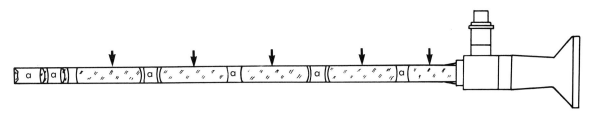

FIG. 2-2 Rod lens system. *a*, Air, *arrows*, lens.

The hysteroscopes most commonly used are 0° straight forward or 30° foreoblique. The angle of view also varies according to the refractory index of the medium used to distend the uterine cavity. The laws of reflection and refraction, by which light projects in a straight line in a medium of uniform index, apply when different distending media are used in hysteroscopy. If a gaseous medium is used the maximal angle of view is perceived through the optic. When a liquid medium is used the angle is reduced.[7]

Several components of the optical system can influence the characteristics of the image, its resolution, contrast, and brightness. Resolution is the ability of an optical instrument to separate the fine detail in an object. Contrast represents the relative difference in intensity between the objects observed and its environment. Details can be seen with good light and diagnoses can be made depending on the ability of the hysteroscopist to evaluate the size, shape, color, and structure of an object.

With the use of fiberoptics, potent light can be transmitted from the source to the hysteroscope without producing excessive heat or breakage of distal bulbs. Thousands of small glass fibers (10 $\mu$) with a high refractory index core and low index cladding, produce a compact system of delivering brighter light efficiently and with minimal loss. These optical components enable the production of high quality, small diameter hysteroscopes that are capable of forming excellent images with wide fields of view.

## Rigid Panoramic Hysteroscopes

Although the basic elements of the cystoscope remain unchanged,[2] the modern hysteroscope, derived from the original cystoscope perfected by McCarthy,[12] has undergone important modifications to adapt its use for the examination of the uterine cavity. Most rigid, fixed focus panoramic hysteroscopes have an outside diameter (OD) of 4 mm with a viewing angle of either 0° (straight on) or 30° (offset) (Fig. 2-3). The telescope with a 4 mm OD, even though narrow, can provide an optimally bright, clear, wide-angle view of an object when combined with a high-intensity light. Selection of a viewing angle is a matter of personal preference. The 30° offset telescope allows observation of the uterine horns and uterotubal ostia when the telescope is rotated to the right or left using the lightpost as a guide. Regardless of whether diagnostic or therapeutic hysteroscopy is contemplated, the OD of the telescope is the same. These instruments are focused at infinity, and therefore, the image is smaller than the actual size when it is positioned away from the object; a meaningful view is obtained when moved closer to the object. It is not possible to measure the precise size of an intrauterine tumor without first knowing the size of another object in the same viewing plane.

Some hysteroscopes can be focused by turning a knob on the proximal end of the endoscope. These models offer panoramic viewing, as well as close-up viewing (see Fig. 2-10, *B*). The gynecologist should check the focusing mechanism on the hysteroscope before inserting it into the endocervical canal to gain perspective. Hysteroscopes are about 30 cm in length with the exception of the microcolpohysteroscope, which is 25 cm long.

One variation of an operative hysteroscope has an offset right angle extension for the ocular lens while the operative channels remain fixed to the straight portion of the scope. This feature permits the introduction of rigid, sturdy instruments with large diameters (Fig. 2-4). It is not popular, since semirigid instruments required in operative hysteroscopy can be delivered through the standard sheaths.

Thinner hysteroscopes have been developed for office use with ODs of 2.7 mm to 3 mm. These hysteroscopes require potent light sources for more illumination to obtain good photographs (Fig. 2-5).

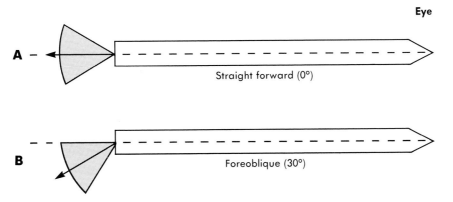

FIG. 2-3 Two common directions of view for hysteroscopes. **A**, Straight forward and **B**, foreoblique. Shaded areas indicate visual field.

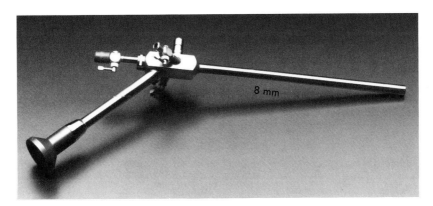

FIG. 2-4 Offset operative hysteroscope has a shaft 8 mm in diameter.

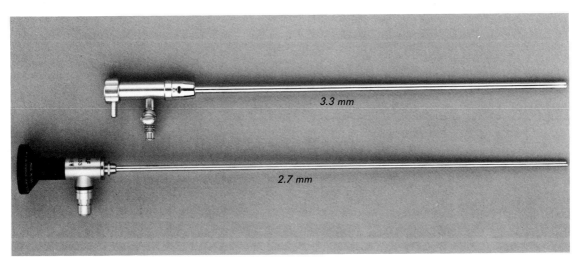

FIG. 2-5 Diagnostic hysteroscope has sheath with OD of 3.3 mm (*top*) and telescope with OD of 2.7 mm (*bottom*).

## Flexible Hysteroscopes

Flexible, steerable, diagnostic hysteroscopes can have an OD of 3.5 mm and are capable of being bent in many directions (Fig. 2-6).[5] The distal tip can be deflected upward or downward at 160° to 130°. The instrument has a 1 mm channel for delivery of distending media.[11] Operative, flexible hysteroscopes with a 4.8 mm OD and an operating channel of 2 mm have been tested. Various accessory instruments can be inserted into the operating channel to remove cornual polyps or adhesions. This instrument offers another alternative for inspection of the lateral areas of the uterine cavity, particularly the uterotubal junctions, in patients with acutely angulated cornua. In these patients, it might be easier to inspect and possibly cannulate the uterotubal ostia. Because it is flexible, this hysteroscope enables the lysis of intrauterine adhesions that are located laterally and difficult to treat by using semirigid scissors introduced through the conventional operative sheath (Figs. 2-7 and 2-8).[20]

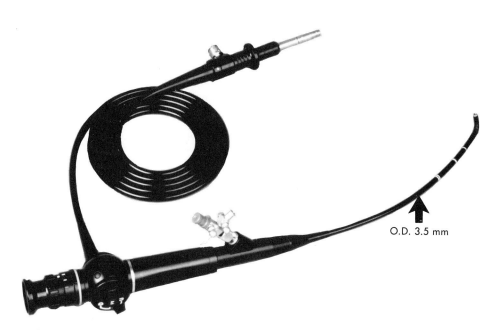

O.D. 3.5 mm

*FIG. 2-6*  Diagnostic hysteroscopic fiberscope has OD of 3.5 mm.

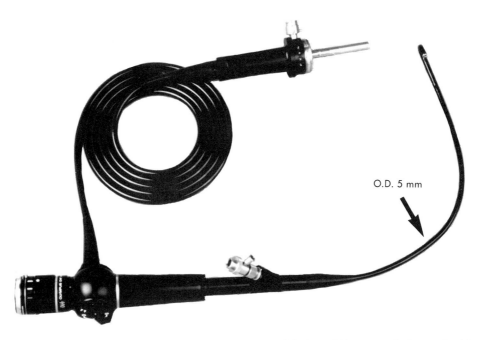

O.D. 5 mm

**FIG. 2-7** Operative hysteroscopic fiberscope with OD of 5 mm and channel with OD of 2 mm for ancillary instruments.

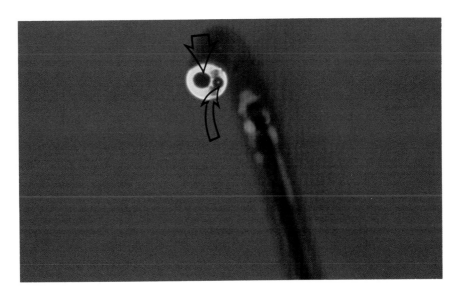

**FIG. 2-8** Closer view of distal end of flexible hysteroscope is shown. Operative channel is 2 mm in diameter (*straight arrow*). Objective lens is indicated by *curved arrow.*

## Contact Hysteroscopes

The contact hysteroscope was introduced as a simple and easy instrument for observing the uterine cavity.[3] The instrument has a transparent solid rod of mineral glass that terminates as a thinly coated, nonreflecting concave mirror. The optical glass is encased in a stainless steel jacket. A cylindrical chamber connected to the glass rod traps ambient light and directs it to the rod by mirrors. The eye-piece has a magnification of 1.6× and the focal length is 4 mm from the surface. This endoscope is available with 4 mm, 6 mm, or 8 mm ODs and has a length of 200 mm. Observations are made only by contact with the surface of the tissue. Since there is no panoramic view, the examination must be performed systematically and progressively to avoid missing areas during the examination. Limited operative procedures can be performed with this instrument, despite attempts to attach a biopsy forceps to the distal end of the sheath (Fig. 2-9). Its best application is exploration of the endocervical canal, particularly as a complement to colposcopy if the lesion extends into the endocervical canal.[1] No distending media are required for contact hysteroscopy. The contact hysteroscope must be held in such a way that nothing obstructs the light collecting chamber. The light source can consist of a room lamp or a special high-intensity halogen lamp. The focusing and magnifying eyepiece can be prefocused on a piece of gauze.

## Microcolpohysteroscope

The microcolpohysteroscope (MCH) is a multipurpose instrument for contact and panoramic hysteroscopy.[8] The telescope has a 4 mm OD, is 25 cm long with a 30° foreoblique view that offers panoramic as well as contact vision at different magnifications (Fig. 2-10). The microcolpohysteroscope set at position 1 offers a conventional panoramic view like the conventional 4 mm hysteroscope. Position 2 is used for close panoramic observation at 20× magnification. Observation is equivalent to that offered by the colposcope. Positions 3 and 4, with magnifications of 60× and 150× respectively, are used for contact observations. Magnifications are used to see the mucosa, glandular structures, papillae, and capillaries. If special stains are used, observations of the nucleus and cytoplasm are possible. When using panoramic hysteroscopes to see details near its distal end and at some distance, it is important not to move the instrument because relative viewing angles and visual magnification change as the instrument is moved. This instrument allows the gynecologist to view the endocervical canal and locate the transformation zone (TZ) within it. The higher magnifications (60× and 150×) require direct application of vital dyes (Lugol's iodine [2%] and a blue ink) to the mucosal surface. After such a preparation, it is possible to observe the pattern of the superficial cellular layers. There is a significant contrast between the immature cells in cervical intraepithelial neoplasia (CIN) and normal mature squamous cells with their large cytoplasm and pyknotic nuclei. It has been suggested that the MCH can be used to locate the area of the TZ where the most abnormal changes are, and therefore, the most appropriate site from which to take the biopsy.

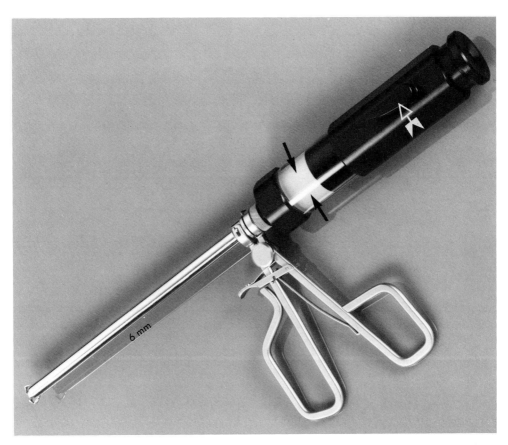

**FIG. 2-9** Contact hysteroscope with distal biopsy forceps attached (Bryan Co.). *Black arrows* indicate collecting light chamber. Lever (*white arrow*) manipulates biopsy forceps.

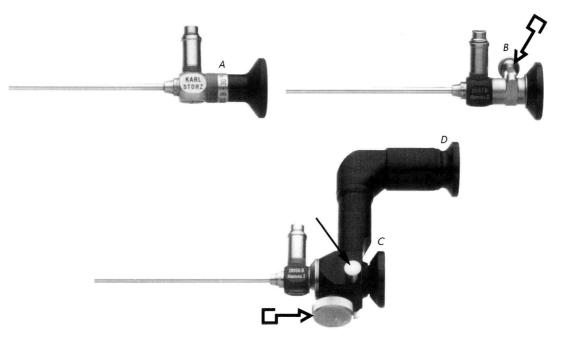

**FIG. 2-10** Standard hysteroscope *A* is 4 mm in diameter and 28 cm long. Focusing hysteroscope *B* has a knob (*arrow*) to adjust focus during entrance of scope through endocervical canal and into uterine cavity. Hamou microcolpohysteroscope *C* has magnifying attachment *D* for contact hysteroscopy. Focusing knob (*broken arrow*) has the same function noted above. *Straight arrow* indicates button that converts view from one ocular lens to other, changing magnifications.

### Portable, Self-contained Hysteroscope

Another type of hysteroscope is a portable, self-contained autonomous unit, providing an endoscopic cold light source and a $CO_2$ insufflator. This compact system is manipulated with one hand and easy to transfer from one location to another. The instrument does not require any external equipment cables or connections, thus offering simplicity and easy maneuverability; storage and cleansing also are facilitated. The instrument was designed by Parent et al.[13] in 1985. The light is provided by a miniature projector equipped with a halogen microlamp that weighs less than 50 g. The projector is connected by a cord to a power source consisting of three rechargeable cadmium-nickel batteries in a case. The case forms the handle used to direct

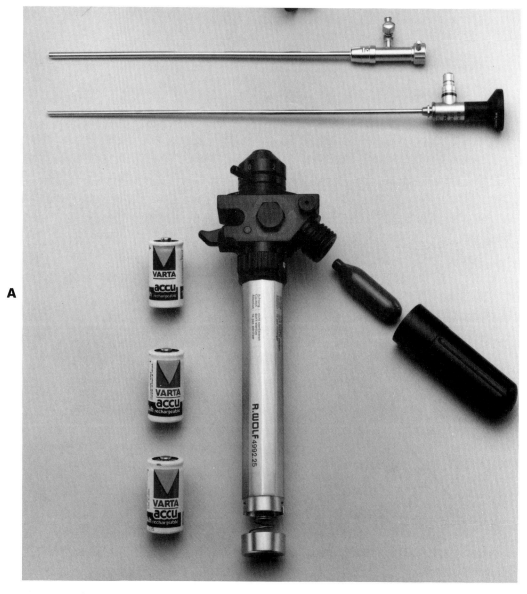

*FIG. 2-11* Components of self-contained automatic hysteroscope. **A,** Telescope and sheath (*top*); portable unit, batteries, and cartridge for $CO_2$ (*bottom*).

the instrument. The batteries provide 1 hour of continuous use and can be recharged with an external charger. Any of the hysteroscopes available for diagnostic purposes or operative intervention can be used. The $CO_2$ gas is provided by a pellet or cartridge that fits laterally into the instrument. The pellet or cartridge contains 4 L of $CO_2$ under pressure and the instrument regulates the pressure of the gas being delivered by rotating a dial from position 0 to position 1 or 2. Position 1 delivers the gas at 75 ml/min with an intrauterine pressure of no more than 75 mm Hg. Position 2 delivers the gas at 100 ml/min with an intrauterine pressure of no more than 150 mm Hg. Each cartridge allows 80 minutes for examinations at a constant flowrate of 50 ml/min. The gas delivery unit has an encased protection valve to allow escape of the gas to prevent excessive pressure, a possible danger for the patient. The advantages of this instrument are ease of manipulation, transport, storage, and care, making it especially suited for an office setting (Fig. 2-11, *A,B*).

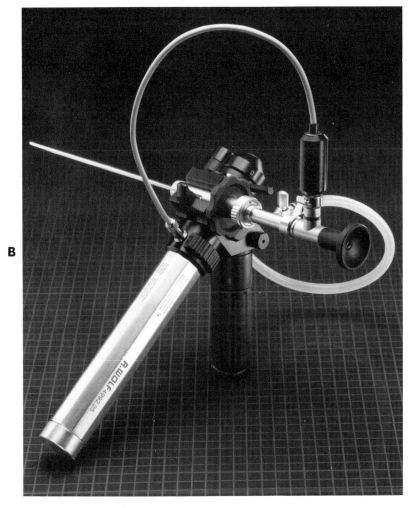

**B**

**FIG. 2-11,** *cont'd*  **B,** Self-contained apparatus has a $CO_2$ cartridge (4 L), a halogen microlamp, and three cadmium-nickel batteries that provide sufficient power for 1 hour. Flowrate is limited to 100 ml/min and cartridge pressure to 150 mm Hg. Insufflator unit cannot be soaked in disinfectant solution or gas sterilized.

## SHEATHS

The hysteroscope is encased in a metallic sheath that is provided in a variety of sizes depending on the need. Operative sheaths are usually 7 mm to 8 mm OD, and diagnostic sheaths are 3.3 mm to 5 mm OD. The sheath is locked in both types to the hysteroscope by turning or clicking the proximal part of the sheath to the hysteroscope (Fig. 2-12). The locking mechanism is an important feature because it must remain fluid or gas tight during an operative procedure. Diagnostic sheaths do not provide channels for accessory instruments but provide only a port for the instillation of the distending medium, usually $CO_2$. The 5 mm diagnostic sheath is suited for an office hysteroscopy when $CO_2$ is used as the distending medium. Instillation of a liquid medium is difficult because of the small space between the juxtaposed endoscope and sheath. It is important that the distal ends of the sheath and endoscope fit exactly so uterine tissue is not inadvertently "scooped" into this space. Also, the gynecologist may wish to withdraw the hysteroscope during an operative procedure but leave the sheath in the uterine cavity. If the locking mechanism is difficult to maneuver, the endometrial surface could be traumatized when the parts are reassembled.

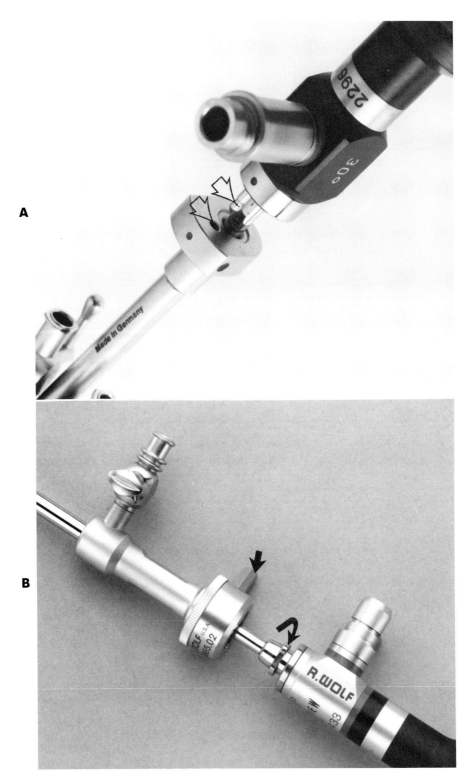

*FIG. 2-12* Different mechanisms show locking of sheath to hysteroscope. **A,** Pin on scope (*arrow*) clicks into hole (*arrow*) on sheath; **B,** thread on scope (*curved arrow*) locks into sheath by turning pin (*straight arrow*).

The operative sheath with the most simple design has stopcocks (right and left) on opposite sides for the instillation of distending media. This arrangement makes it difficult to irrigate the uterine cavity by injecting through one channel while leaving the other open. An operating channel on the posterior surface of the sheath is fitted with a rubber nipple to prevent loss of the medium while accessory instruments are being maneuvered (Fig. 2-13).

Contemporary designs have double ports that are isolated from each other and allow rinsing of the uterine cavity. Continuous irrigation is especially important with laser and resectoscopic surgery. Inflow and outflow channels allow removal of blood clots, debris, and tissue fragments that tend to cloud distending media.

A third channel is used to instill the distending medium and a fourth one is used for the insertion of accessory instruments. The distal end of another sheath that was designed by Baggish is shown (Fig. 2-14). The distal lens of the hysteroscope is flush with the end of the sheath and two other ports can be used interchangeably for manipulating two accessory instruments or for irrigating the uterine cavity. The remaining channel is used to instill the distending medium. This arrangement permits irrigating and operating simultaneously.

An Albarran elevator (bridge) or deflecting mechanism, similar to the one found on the operating cystoscope, is useful with flexible instruments, catheters, or laser fibers (see Fig. 2-17). This deflecting mechanism is guided by a small lever attached to the proximal part of the sheath. It allows the gynecologist to guide accessory instruments to the area of interest and converts the flexible instrument into a semirigid one.[2] It is most useful for operative procedures involving the cornua and uterotubal ostia.

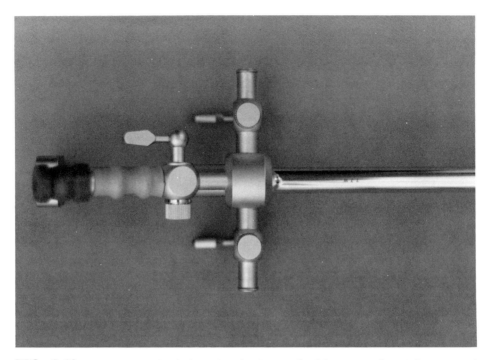

*FIG. 2-13* Proximal end of this sheath shows double stopcocks, either one of which can be used to instill medium. Port on posterior aspect is channel for insertion of 7 Fr semirigid biopsy or grasping forceps and scissors.

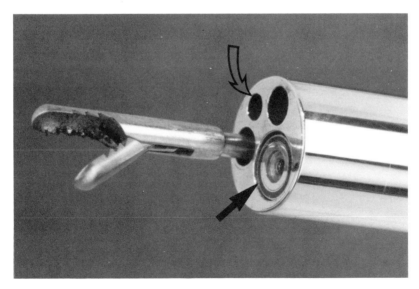

*FIG. 2-14* Distal end of sheath has four openings. Objective lens of hysteroscope (*straight arrow*) is in one, grasping forceps protrude from another, medium comes from third (*curved arrow*), and another accessory instrument can project from fourth opening (Bryon Co.).

Some operative sheaths have a removable obturator for easier introduction of the hysteroscope through the endocervical canal. Sheaths have beveled ends and can be used as obturators.[18] Another type of sheath contains an operating instrument (scissors or biopsy forceps) attached to the distal end. Although this feature permits easier and faster division of thick intrauterine adhesions, septa, or resection of submucous myomas, its use requires special attention. Since the tip of the forceps remains fixed to the sheath, care should be taken to achieve a clear panoramic view of the uterine cavity to avoid perforation (Fig. 2-15) (Table 2-1).

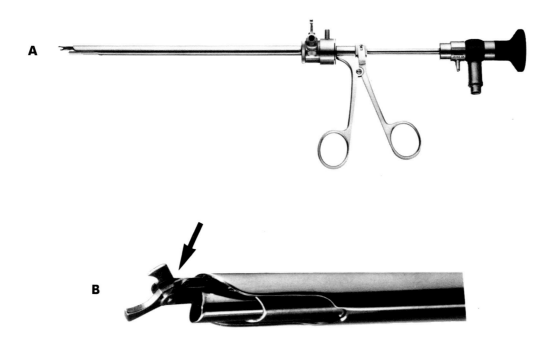

FIG. 2-15 **A,** Fixed, rigid scissors are shown at distal end of sheath with hysteroscope in place. **B,** Closer view of end of sheath with scissors (*arrow*) and end of hysteroscope under it.

*Table 2-1* Characteristics of Operative Sheaths and Accessory Instruments

| Manufacturer* | Sheath Diameter (mm OD) | Inflow-Outflow Irrigation | Obturator Insertion | Accessory Instruments | | |
|---|---|---|---|---|---|---|
| | | | | Flexible | Semirigid | Rigid |
| Bryan | 8 | + | − | + | + | − |
| Eder | 6.2 | + | − | + | + | − |
| Elmed | 7 | − | − | + | − | − |
| Euro-Med | 7.8 | + | − | + | + | − |
| Machida | 7 | + | + | + | − | − |
| Olympus | 7 | ± | − | + | + | + |
| Storz | 7 | ± | + | + | + | + |
| Wisap | 7 | − | − | + | − | − |
| Wolf | 7 | ± | + | + | + | + |

*All telescopes have 0° or 30° angle of view; Olympus also has a 12° hysteroscope.

## RESECTOSCOPES

The urologic resectoscope has been adapted for use in hysteroscopy for the removal of submucous leiomyomas and endometrial polyps, resection of uterine septa, division of thick, connective tissue intrauterine adhesions, and ablation of the endometrium.

The resectoscope includes either a 0° or 30° telescope with a 4 mm OD that can be encased in different sheaths from 6 mm to 8 mm OD (24 Fr to 28 Fr) and each has an appropriate cutting loop. The resectoscope has a spring handle that moves the right-angled wire loop in and out of the distal end of the sheath to electrosurgically shave, resect, or coagulate lesions (Fig. 2-16). The loops are color coded yellow, white, or blue, and each one is used with its appropriate sheath. After the sheath and its obturator have been inserted into the endometrial cavity, the obturator is withdrawn and the loop and telescope mounted in the working elements are substituted. The loop is moved in and out of the sheath so that the position can be observed before being connected to a high frequency electrosurgical unit; proper grounding of the patient is essential. An electrolyte-free solution should be used for distention of the uterine cavity to avoid conduction.

The sheath provides inflow and outflow channels for continuous irrigation. It also permits the introduction of instruments for biopsy or injection of solutions after replacing the cutting loop. The right angled cutting loop can be moved about 3 cm within the visual field of the objective lens. A clear, unobstructed, panoramic view of the lesion and its surrounding normal endometrium is essential. Resectoscopes manufactured by several companies have similar features with minor modifications.

The resecting loop is activated only as it is being drawn into the sheath under direct vision. Sometimes resected tissue tends to float in the endometrial cavity or adheres to the wire loop, obscuring the surgeon's view. The resectoscope should be removed and the sheath left in situ so debris can be removed and the loop cleaned. Recent technical innovations permit electronically controlled irrigation of the uterus when liquid media is used during the operative procedure. The liquid medium flows at 50 ml/min to 200 ml/min at a safe low pressure below 50 mm Hg. When combined with a high frequency electrosurgical unit, the system provides a predictable, rapid, and unobscured view during the entire operation. It is essential that the hysteroscopist has experience doing diagnostic procedures and simpler therapeutic maneuvers before doing complicated procedures, especially when the resectoscope is used. Collaboration with the urologist for the initial procedures which involve the use of this instrument can be quite helpful and reassuring.

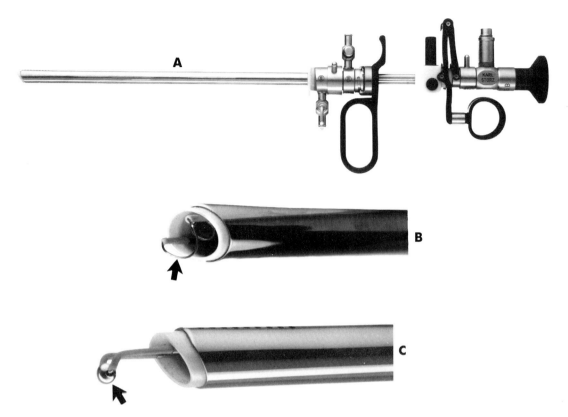

*FIG. 2-16* **A,** Resectoscope assembled. **B,** Close-up view of distal end of resecto-scope shows cutting loop *(arrow).* **C,** Roller ball *(arrow)* has been attached to resec-toscope for coagulation and endometrial ablation procedure.

## LASERS

Laser is an acronym for *L*ight *A*mplification of *S*timulated *E*mission of *R*adiation. Each laser has specific properties for delivery, effect on tissues (coagulation/vaporization), penetration, scatter, and interaction with different media depending on the power output and wavelength (Table 2-2). Laser operations require manual dexterity, especially hand, eye, and foot coordination. Since laser beams travel at the speed of light, response to activation is instantaneous and accurate. Several surgical lasers are available for hysteroscopic use. Each laser has different properties with advantages and disadvantages in the treatment of intrauterine abnormalities.

The $CO_2$ laser has been the most widely used laser in gynecology, but its endoscopic use has been limited to laparoscopy. Lasers capable of being delivered through fiberoptics are being used with hysteroscopy. In particular, the neodymium-yttrium-aluminum-garnet (Nd:YAG) is being used for the ablation of the endometrium. The beam of the Nd:YAG is invisible (near infrared 1064 nm) and therefore has to be guided by a helium-neon spot. The Nd:YAG wave penetrates deeply into tissue and exerts its major action beneath the tissue target. It is absorbed by tissue protein, penetrates the tissue 3 mm or 4 mm in depth, and its principal effect is photocoagulation rather than vaporization. Since the wave can be transmitted through fiberoptics, it is easily delivered through the operating channel of the hysteroscope with a 0.6 mm diameter quartz fiber. This laser is poorly absorbed by water and therefore penetrates liquid media; it is equally effective on all colors of tissue. Sapphire tips for the Nd:YAG laser enable direct contact (touch technique) and allow the gynecologist to manipulate structures as one does using electrosurgical devices or a scalpel. Because of backscattering, the gynecologist needs the protection of a safety filter on the eyepiece of the hysteroscope or tinted goggles to avoid retinal injury. The Nd:YAG laser requires special wiring, transformers, and plumbing for cooling.

*Table 2-2* Physical Properties of Lasers Used in Hysteroscopic Surgery

| Type | Wavelength (nm) | Color Spectrum | Power (w) | Absorption | Aiming Beam |
|---|---|---|---|---|---|
| Argon | 488-512 | Blue-green | 0-20 | Hemoglobin | Argon |
| KTP/532 | 532 | Green | 0-40 | Hemoglobin | KTP |
| Nd:YAG | 1,064 | Near infrared | 0-170 | Tissue protein | Helium-neon |
| $CO_2$ | 10,600 | Near infrared | 0-100* | Fluids | Helium-neon |

*Superpulse mode has a maximal peak power from 500 to 5,000 w. *nm*, Nanometers; *w*, watts.

## Laser Terminology

**ablation**   volume removal of tissue by vaporization.

**aiming beam**   a HeNe laser (or other light source) used as a guide light coaxially with infrared or other invisible light.

**argon**   the gas used as a laser medium that emits blue-green light at 488 and 512 nm.

**carbon dioxide**   the gas used as a laser medium that emits infrared light at 10,600 nm.

**coagulation**   destruction of tissue by heat without physically removing it.

**coherence**   wave patterns that are in phase in time and space.

**collimation**   ability of laser beam not to diverge and remain parallel with distance.

**contact probe**   a synthetic ceramic material (sapphire) used with laser fibers to enable touching of the tissue with the laser probe. The effects are intensified so that cutting, vaporizing, or tissue coagulation become feasible at relatively low powers with good control.

**continuous wave**   constant, steady state delivery of laser power.

**electromagnetic spectrum**   the span of wavelengths of light (frequencies) from radio and television waves to gamma and cosmic rays.

**fiberoptics**   flexible quartz or glass fibers with internal reflective surfaces that pass light through hundreds of thousands of fibers to transmit an image. Only a single fiber is needed to transmit laser light.

**Gaussian curve**   used to show power distribution in a beam that is like a normal statistical bell-shaped curve showing a peak with an even distribution on either side. It may be either a sharp peak with steep sides or a blunt peak with shallow sides.

**HeNe**   a low power (milliwatts) laser red light (630 nm) used as a guide light for infrared lasers.

**joule**   laser power is sometimes described in joules (a unit of energy) per second. A power of one joule per second is known as one watt and is the amount of energy delivered.

**KTP**   potassium titanyl phosphate is a crystal used to change the wavelength of Nd:YAG laser from 1060 nm (infrared) to 532 nm (green).

**laser**   light amplication by the stimulated emission of radiation. A device that produces intense beams of pure colors of light.

**laser medium**   material used to emit laser light from which the laser is named.

**monochromaticity**   waves of all the same color (wavelength).

**nanometer**   nm is used to measure the light wavelength. Visible light ranges from about 400 nm in the purple to about 750 nm in the deep red.

**neodymium**   the rare earth element that is the active element in a Nd:YAG laser.

**power density**   the amount of energy concentrated into a spot of a particular size. It is expressed in watts per square centimeter and is the brightness of the spot.

**pulse**   a burst of laser energy as compared to a continuous beam. A true pulse achieves higher peak power than is attainable in a continuous wave output.

**spot size**   the optical spot size and not necessarily the size of the laser crater (the impact size). It is the mathematical measurement of the focused laser spot. In a TEMoo beam, it contains 86% of the incident power.

Other lasers under investigation for hysteroscopic application are the potassium-titanyl-phosphate (KTP/532) and the argon lasers. The argon laser emits in the blue-green wavelength (532 nm) of the electromagnetic spectrum (visible). Tinted goggles or a safety filter over the eyepiece of the hysteroscope must be worn for eye protection. The argon laser also can be transmitted by fine flexible quartz fibers, but it has a very low power compared to Nd:YAG or the $CO_2$ lasers. An 8 to 14 watt setting is used with a 2 mm spot size and a 2 to 5 second delivery time. The laser energy generated with the KTP/532 can pass through a flexible quartz fiber with up to 12 watts of energy available to the tissue. The depth of tissue penetration (about 3 mm) of the KTP/532 laser is similar to that of the argon laser but less than the Nd:YAG laser. These three lasers have flexible fiberoptics with a capability for energy to be transmitted through water, eliminating the need to work in a dry field. In addition, argon and KTP/532 lasers produce less smoke than the $CO_2$ laser, a feature that helps keep the gynecologist's line of vision clear. The energy of argon lasers is absorbed selectively by hemosiderin. The KTP/532 and argon lasers are coagulating lasers. To operate the KTP/532, argon, or Nd:YAG lasers, the gynecologist must use either a monoshutter and miniature hysteroscopic mounted video camera, a video recorder and a high resolution video monitor, or protective tinted goggles. The flexible fibers of the argon and KTP/532 lasers break or melt at high wattage settings but even settings as low as 8 to 12 watts can destroy them.

The fiber guide for the $CO_2$ laser perhaps can be a good addition for the hysteroscopist treating intrauterine lesions without the backscattering and penetration expected from the Nd:YAG. However the laser smoke (plume) caused by explosive evaporation (vaporization) must be removed and this maneuver results in the loss of uterine distention. Ideally the tunable free-electron lasers may profoundly change the clinical applications of laser energy by allowing the delivery of coherent radiation over a broad range of wavelengths from the far infrared to the far ultraviolet regions of the spectrum.[4]

In selecting a specific laser for intrauterine surgery the features pertinent to each laser should be considered: penetration, scattering, absorption in the distending medium, power, portability, as well as the surgical objectives (Table 2-3).

Because of bubbling of the medium or formation of debris, the capability to rinse the uterine cavity is required when the intrauterine laser is used. This can be accomplished by using sheaths with inflow and outflow channels. Intrauterine laser procedures sometimes can be prolonged and require large volumes of distending media. It is important to use fluids containing electrolytes (they will not interfere with the delivery of the laser) and to measure carefully the volume used (input and output) to prevent water overload and the occurrence of noncardiogenic pulmonary edema.

*Table 2-3*  Clinical Features of Lasers Used for Hysteroscopic Surgery

| Type | Flexible Fiber | Scattering of Beam | Absorption by Fluid | Depth of Penetration | Primary Effect | |
|------|----------------|--------------------|--------------------|----------------------|-----------------|------------|
| | | | | | Coagulation | Vaporization |
| Argon | Yes | Slight | No | 1 mm | Yes | Slight |
| KTP/532 | Yes | Slight | No | 1-2 mm | Yes | Slight |
| Nd:YAG | Yes | Significant* | No | 3-4 mm | Significant | Slight |
| | | | | | | Significant with sapphire tip† |
| $CO_2$ | Yes | None | Significant | >1 mm‡ | Minimal | Significant |

*Forward and back scatter.
†Absorbs energy and controls depth of penetration.
‡Depth of penetration readily controlled.

## LIGHT SOURCES AND CABLES

Light cables are flexible bundles of glass fibers that transmit the light from an external source to the endoscope and snap securely into the lightpost of the endoscope. Most manufacturers provide special adapters to allow interchanging light sources and cables. Fiberoptic cables are about 3.5 mm to 4.4 mm OD with a length of about 200 cm. A special fluid-filled light cable, with an OD of 3 mm and 180 cm in length, has been advocated for photography because this cable's transmission of light was presumed to be more efficient than transmission obtained through conventional glass bundles. This cable is less flexible and should not be bent in a short radius. Some light cables are integrated with endoscopes to avoid the loss of light that occurs at the interface of the standard connection. Such cables are not practical because their manipulation and cleaning are difficult; they are seldom used with hysteroscopes, except in special flexible ones.

Other light sources available for endoscopic procedures can be used for hysteroscopy including those containing a 150 watt lamp, and small portable units with or without flash generators. Most of these units are useful for diagnostic and therapeutic procedures.

For cinematography or video recording, the xenon light source with a color-corrected temperature of 5,400° to 6,000° is required. Flash generators are available from most manufacturers and are essential for production of high-quality still pictures.[19]

## ACCESSORY INSTRUMENTS FOR HYSTEROSCOPY

A variety of flexible, rigid, and semirigid instruments have been designed for use in hysteroscopic surgery. The flexible and semirigid instruments can be inserted through a channel in the sheath for intrauterine surgery (Fig. 2-17). The Albarran bridge converts the flexible instruments into semirigid ones. These instruments include grasping forceps, biopsy forceps, and scissors. Some operative instruments are attached to the end of the sheath and must be maneuvered with the hysteroscope for proper use. The flexible and semi-rigid instruments are 7 Fr. The semirigid instruments are preferred by most hysteroscopists and are useful for cutting septa and intrauterine adhesions. These instruments, the biopsy and grasping forceps, and scissors, are very delicate. A shaft or handle can be destroyed by rough manipulation. When-ever Hyskon is used as the distending medium, the instruments must be carefully rinsed in hot water to prevent the jaws of the instrument from adhering to each other.

The rigid accessory instruments can be inserted through an offset oper-ating hysteroscope (see Fig. 2-4), which has a shaft OD of 8 mm. However they are more difficult to maneuver than the semirigid forceps and scissors. The other type of rigid operating instrument has either the scissors or biopsy forceps fixed to the end of the metal sheath (see Fig. 2-15).

Catheters made of plastic tubing are used to irrigate the uterine cavity to remove blood clots, mucus, and debris (Fig. 2-18). The lumen of these cathe-ters should be wide enough to allow this flushing effect and not become plugged; they should be stiff enough so they can be inserted easily through one of the channels on the sheath. The internal diameter (ID) of such a catheter is about 1.7 mm and the OD is 2.3 mm. A 15-gauge needle or adapter, attached to a syringe, can be placed at one end for irrigation and suction. As liquids are injected through these catheters, the ends can be moved back and forth independently of the optical system. This technique can allow the physician to change a cloudy operative field into a clear one and to reduce the incidence of inadvertent trauma to the uterine wall, which happens when the physician is unable to see the relationship of the operat-ing instruments to the uterine abnormality.

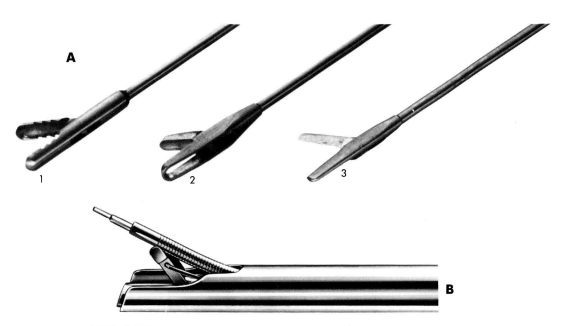

FIG. 2-17  **A,** Distal ends of grasping forceps (*1*), biopsy forceps (*2*), and scissors (*3*) are shown. **B,** Albarran bridge bends tip of flexible instrument.

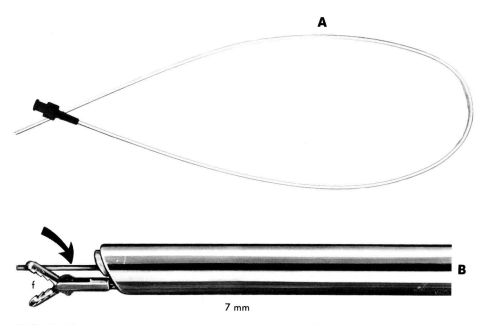

FIG. 2-18  **A,** Aspiration catheters are about 7 Fr (2.3 mm OD) and have Luer adaptor at one end. **B,** Catheter (*arrow*) is used for flushing and aspirating debris and blood clots during operative hysteroscopy. Grasping forcep (*f*) is seen *below.*

## ANESTHESIA

Pain relief must be appropriate for the type of hysteroscopic examination and be the desire and choice of the patient. Endotracheal intubation has become the most widely accepted method of administering general anesthesia for laparoscopy. Local anesthesia used alone or in combination with systemic analgesia is sufficient for most hysteroscopic examinations. These are administered by the endoscopist; the equipment and drugs to treat complications must be available. Patients should be asked about any previous reactions to local anesthesia. Skill and gentle handling can prevent some adverse reactions. The minimal effective dose and concentration of the agent should be used, making sure to wait long enough for the anesthetic to take effect. When administered as a paracervical block, the injection should be interrupted for intermittent aspiration to detect vascular intravasation. Continuous conversation with the patient can reassure her and help detect toxic manifestations. Adverse systemic reactions principally affect the central nervous system. Patients may become light-headed and drowsy and have blurred vision, but reactions are usually mild and short. Such complaints are the result of high plasma levels caused by rapid absorption, an inadvertent intravascular injection, or an excessive dosage. Other causes include hypersensitivity, idiosyncrasy, or decreased tolerance.

Hysteroscopy requires the use of a tenaculum on the anterior lip of the cervix that can cause pain for some patients and indicates a need for local anesthesia or analgesia. For diagnostic office examinations, no more than 20% of women who have been pregnant need pain relief during the procedure. When small caliber sheaths (about 5 mm OD) are used for diagnostic purposes, mild sedation or 10 ml of a local anesthetic such as lidocaine 1% without epinephrine can be injected either paracervically or into the vaginal mucous membrane beneath the posterior lip of the cervix. Some gynecologists choose to infiltrate the cervix at four sites instead. These short-acting agents have a low toxicity. If cervical dilatation becomes a part of the procedure, local anesthesia is essential. The procedure should be explained to the patient preoperatively, preferably using a pamphlet that includes the indications for the operation, a simplified explanation of the technique, aftereffects, risks, and the possible need of a hospital-based hysteroscopic examination.

Cervical dilatation often becomes necessary when hysteroscopy is performed using operative sheaths. A paracervical block is required for removal of IUDs; biopsy of lesions; division of small, focal, filmy, intrauterine adhesions; and sterilization with intratubal devices. General anesthesia administered by endotracheal intubation is used, if hysteroscopy is performed concomitantly with laparoscopy and during hysteroscopic lysis of severe (Stage 3) intrauterine adhesions, removal of submucous leiomyomas, and hysteroscopic metroplasty. Epidural anesthesia is effective for prolonged hysteroscopic operations (i.e., endometrial ablation) or when general anesthesia is contraindicated.

Local anesthesia and general anesthesia did not appear to cause any clinically significant change in acid-base balance according to Salat-Baroux et al.[17] who measured arterial blood gases during different anesthetic techniques and used three types of media to distend the uterine cavity. The least alterations in blood gases were the result of carbon dioxide insufflation at a fixed rate of 30 ml/min with variable pressures and anesthesia. An endotracheal tube was rarely needed to maintain controlled respirations.

**SUMMARY**

Attention to details of the characteristics and maintenance of the instruments described in this chapter will increase success with their use and increase the confidence of the gynecologist. Most of the technical problems with the equipment that can happen during hysteroscopic operations can be located and corrected.

*References*

1. Baggish MS: Contact hysteroscopy: a new technique to explore the uterine cavity, Obstet Gynecol 54:350, 1977.
2. Baggish MS: New instruments and techniques for hysteroscopy, Contemp Obstet Gynecol 22:67, 1984.
3. Barbot J, Parent B, and Dubuisson JB: Contact hysteroscopy: another method of endoscopic examination of the uterine cavity, Am J Obstet Gynecol 136:721, 1980.
4. Brau CA: Free electron lasers, Science 239:1115, 1988.
5. Brueschke EE and Wilbanks GD: A steerable fiberoptic hysteroscope, Obstet Gynecol 44:273, 1974.
6. Epstein M: Endoscopy: developments in optical instrumentation, Science 210:280, 1980.
7. Gardner FM: Optical physics with emphasis on endoscope, Clin Obstet Gynecol 26:213, 1983.
8. Hamou J: Microhysteroscopy: a new procedure and its original applications in gynecology, J Reprod Med 26:375, 1981.
9. Hopkins HH: Optical principles of the endoscope. In Berci G, ed: Endoscopy. New York, 1976, Appleton-Century-Crofts.
10. Hopkins HH: Physics of the fiberoptic endoscope. In Berci G, ed: New York, 1976, Appleton-Century-Crofts.
11. Lin BL, Miyamoto N, Tomatsu M, et al.: Flexible hysterofiberscope. The development of a new flexible hysterofiberscope and its clinical application, Acta Obstet Gynecol Jap 39:649, 1987.
12. McCarthy JF: A new type observation and operating cystourethroscope, J Urol 10:519, 1923.
13. Parent B, Guedj H, Barbot J, et al.: Panoramic hysteroscopy, Baltimore, 1987, Williams & Wilkins.
14. Prescott R: Optical principles of endoscopy, J Med Primatol 5:133, 1976.
15. Quint RH: The rigid hysteroscope. In Sciarra JJ, Butler JC, and Speidel JJ, eds: Hysteroscopic sterilization, New York, 1974, Intercontinental Medical Book Corp.
16. Quint RH: Physics of light and image transmission. In Phillips JP, Corson SL, Keith L, et al., eds: Laparoscopy, Baltimore, 1977, Williams & Wilkins.
17. Salat-Baroux J, Hamou JE, Maillard G, et al.: Complications from microhysteroscopy. In Siegler AM and Lindemann HJ, eds: Hysteroscopy: principles and practice, Philadelphia, 1984, JB Lippincott.
18. Valle RF and Sciarra JJ: Current status of hysteroscopy in gynecologic practice, Fertil Steril 32:619, 1979.
19. Valle RF: Hysteroscopy for gynecologic diagnosis, Clin Obstet Gynecol 26:253, 1983.
20. Valle RF: Future growth and development of hysteroscopy, Obstet Gynecol Clin No Am 15:111, 1988.

# 3 *Media*

The uterine cavity is a potential space that is accessible after traversing the cervical canal. To provide a panoramic view for the examiner, the cavity must be distended. It must be illuminated to allow inspection, to attain a targeted biopsy, and to perform a therapeutic operative procedure.

Although the choice of medium is often arbitrary, the agent used must sufficiently distend the uterine cavity to allow adequate observation during the operative procedure, minimize uterine bleeding by creating a sustained intrauterine pressure, and not interfere with the therapeutic technique. Attempting a hysteroscopic examination without distending the uterine cavity would be like performing a laparoscopy without pneumoperitoneum. The most commonly used media are carbon dioxide, low viscosity fluids, and high molecular weight dextran 70.[18]

## CARBON DIOXIDE

$CO_2$ has a refractive index of 1.00 that allows excellent observation and facilitates the development of high quality photographs. $CO_2$ requires a special insufflator that limits the flowrate to not more than 100 ml/min and the intrauterine pressure to 200 mm Hg, and has a reducing valve that ensures the accuracy of the flowrate. If the tubes are closed, as the intrauterine pressure approaches 200 mm Hg, the flowrate automatically decreases to 0. In patients who have patent tubes the $CO_2$ flowrate is between 40 and 60 ml/min with an average intrauterine pressure of 60 to 80 mm Hg.

Two types of hysteroscopic insufflators are currently used. In one the pressure is set to 100 mm Hg, and $CO_2$ is instilled until the preset pressure has been reached (Fig. 3-1, *A*).[17] With the second type of insufflator, the flowrate is preset and as the intrauterine pressure rises, the flowrate falls automatically (Fig. 3-1, *B*).

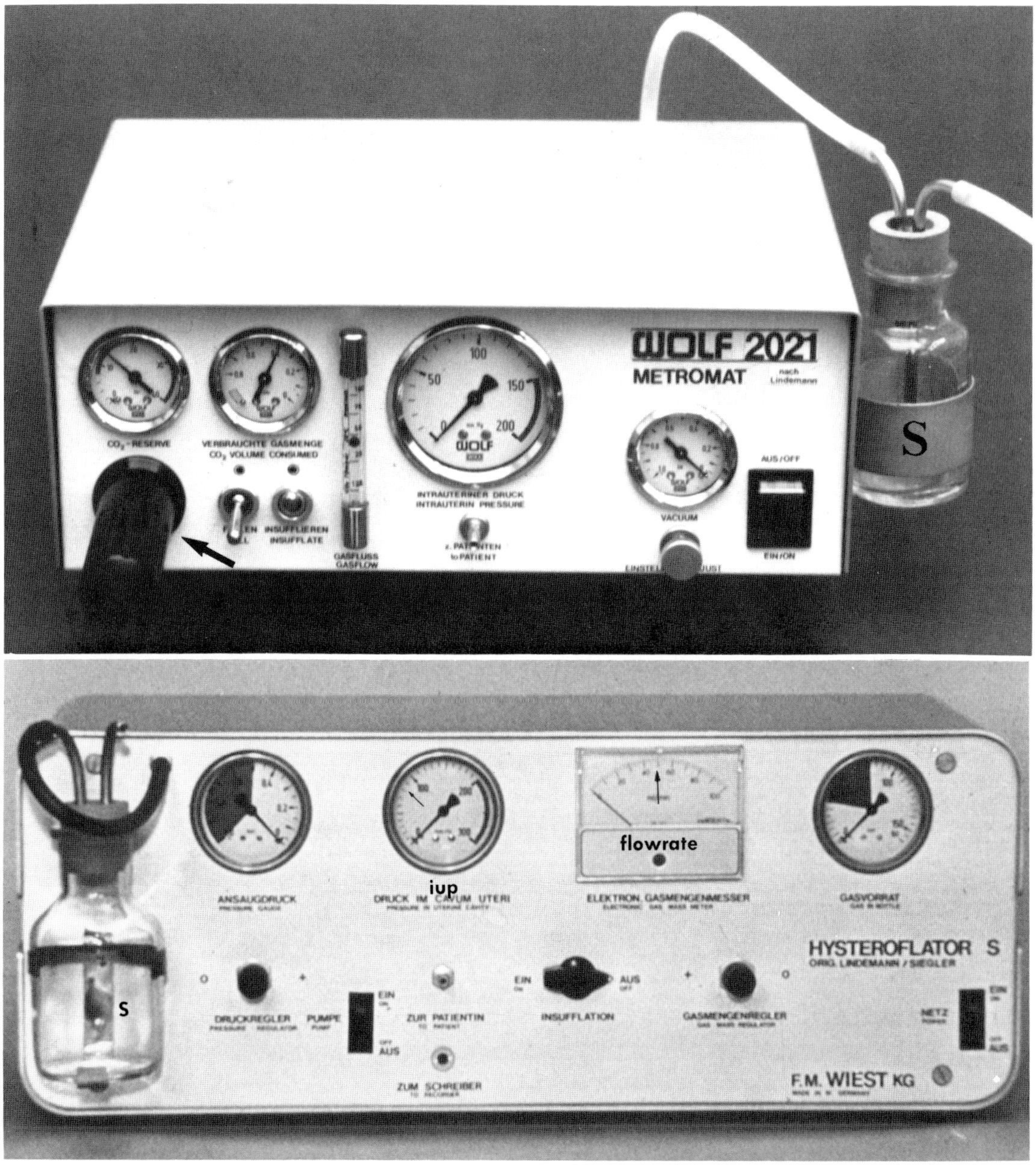

FIG. 3-1  A, With CO$_2$ insufflator, pressure is preset and gas flows until set pressure is reached. *Arrow* indicates CO$_2$ cartridge. B, With this insufflator, flowrate (*long arrow*) is set between 40 and 60 ml/min. With normally patent tubes average intra-uterine pressure remains between 60 and 80 mm Hg (*short arrow*). Glass bottles (*S*) are used with cervical suction cups.

If the view is obscured and the pressure is very low (less than 10 mm Hg), despite a high flowrate (more than 80 ml/min), a leak in the system or uterine perforation should be suspected. Bubbles of mucus and bleeding during intrauterine operations can make observation of the contours of the cavity difficult or impossible. Suction or irrigation often helps to overcome these problems. Superficial, capillary bleeding usually stops with intrauterine pressures of 100 mm Hg. Postoperative shoulder pain can be prevented by arranging the examination table in a slight Trendelenburg position for about 10 to 15 minutes after the examination.

The advantages of using $CO_2$ are the near-perfect transmission of the image, availability, a long history of safety in tubal patency testing, rapid absorption, and ease of cleaning instruments postoperatively. The volume of $CO_2$ required for any procedure is not significant. The insufflator used for laparoscopy should never be used for $CO_2$ hysteroscopy because it has a flowrate of at least 1 L per minute.

Disadvantages of using $CO_2$ for hysteroscopy include requiring a special insufflating apparatus, taking extreme care to avoid gas bubbles and mucus or blood, and maintaining distention of the uterine cavity, despite the escape of gas through patent tubes or a patulous cervix (Table 3-1).

*Table 3-1*  Carbon Dioxide Distending Medium

| Advantages | Disadvantages |
|---|---|
| Excellent image, refractive index 1.00 | Special insufflator essential to limit rate of flow |
| Rapid absorption | |
| Volume of gas used unimportant | Gas bubbles annoying |
| Long history of safety | Less than ideal for operative hysteroscopy |
| Ideal for office hysteroscopy | Difficult to use with laser (plume evacuation) |

## TECHNIQUES OF OFFICE HYSTEROSCOPY USING CO$_2$

For diagnostic purposes, hysteroscopy can be performed in the office using CO$_2$ to distend the uterine cavity.[3,19] In most patients, a hysteroscope with a 5 mm OD sheath can be introduced into the uterine cavity without the need for either a paracervical block or analgesia. Whenever a local anesthetic is required, it can be administered by injecting about 10 ml of an appropriate drug into the vaginal mucous membrane beneath the cervix to create a wheal.

The principles of this technique include a preliminary pelvic examination to ascertain the uterine position and size, and a review of the patient's history and previous hysterosalpingogram to alert the physician to specific defects. The speculum should be unhinged on one side to enable greater manipulation of the hysteroscope. A tenaculum is placed on the anterior lip of the cervix for traction. The patient's buttocks are elevated about 15°, the CO$_2$ flowrate and fiberoptic light projector are adjusted, and their connections are attached to the appropriate places on the sheath and hysteroscope.

The flowrate of CO$_2$ is set between 40 to 60 ml/min and should remain constant, depending on the resistance at the uterotubal junctions. Occluded tubes cause the pressure to rise to 200 mm Hg as the flowrate falls to 0. The arrangement between flowrate and pressure is an important safety feature. Some CO$_2$ does escape the external os but it is not sufficient to prevent adequate, sustained dilatation of the uterine cavity. No cervical cap or occlusive device is required to prevent escape of the gas, and leakage at the cervix usually can be prevented by adjusting the tenaculum to narrow the os. The tip of the hysteroscope and its sheath are inserted gently into the cervical canal, while the surgeon observes through the panoramic ocular lens. As the endocervix fills, its projections can be seen clearly within the canal during dilatation, using CO$_2$. Slow rotation of the hysteroscope often facilitates its passage, but usually some resistance is encountered just before the uterine cavity is entered. The gynecologist is ready to explore the fundus systematically: both uterine horns and ostia and the lateral, anterior, and posterior walls of the uterine cavity. When a normal cavity distends, the endometrium appears pale yellow, tan, or pink with occasional hemorrhagic spots.

When learning to do diagnostic hysteroscopy, the proliferative phase should be selected for easiest interpretation. The proliferative endometrium is thin, while the secretory endometrium is thicker; the depth of the endometrium can be estimated after penetrating it with the end of the hysteroscope. Since the endometrial surfaces are fairly close together, the hysteroscope must be rotated carefully to explore the entire cavity. The uterotubal junctions can be located by gently manipulating the instrument until the uterine horn comes into view, the tubal ostia will be at the apex. Frequently the cavity, both uterine horns, and ostia can be seen simultaneously. The hysteroscope is slowly withdrawn to reinspect the isthmic and endocervical canals. Following their removal, the hysteroscope and its sheath are cleaned and irrigated with a disinfectant solution. Most studies are completed within 5 minutes so that rarely more than 250 ml of CO$_2$ are used.

**Potential Problems**

1. *Pain.*

   Use 10 ml of 1% lidocaine without epinephrine and inject it into the vaginal mucous membrane beneath the cervix to create a wheal. Use a 25-gauge needle on a needle extender or a tonsil needle (Fig. 3-2). In most instances, even in patients not previously pregnant, a hysteroscope with a sheath with an OD that measures slightly over 5 mm can be introduced into the uterine cavity without the need for either a local anesthetic or analgesia. Although there is some discomfort for the patient as the hysteroscope passes through the lower uterine segment, no medication is required for relief of pain in over 80% of patients.

2. *The cervical canal is narrow.*

   If the hysteroscope and sheath do not pass easily, check the precise course of the uterine cavity with a uterine sound. Gently dilate the canal to 5 mm and then reinsert the instrument. Avoid excessive cervical dilatation, since the canal can become too patulous and maintaining uterine distension could be a problem.

3. *The "black area" in the canal is not seen.*

   This dark area in the background represents the fundus and it should be visible at the 6 o'clock position (Fig. 3-3). As the gynecologist moves the instrument toward this area, the cavity comes into view (Fig. 3-4). If this dark area is not apparent, manipulate the hysteroscope slowly because a 30° angled lens sometimes can be misleading in indicating the direction for advancement of the instrument.

4. *No intrauterine pressure is recorded on the insufflating apparatus.*

   Check the connections to the sheath, those between the sheath, and the hysteroscope to be sure they are fastened securely; readjust to be certain.

5. *Blood obscures the landmarks within the cavity.*

   Never advance the hysteroscope in a cloudy field or in a cavity that is not distended. Observe the insufflating apparatus and note the flowrate of $CO_2$; the intrauterine pressure should be at least 30 mm Hg. Although mucosal bleeding occasionally occurs during manipulation, it rarely prevents adequate observation. The amount of intrauterine pressure developed during instillation of the media helps reduce bleeding. Biopsy under vision causes minimal bleeding, and even following curettage for nonobstetric bleeding, adequate hysteroscopic observations are possible.

6. *The uterotubal ostia are not seen.*

   Slowly rotate the hysteroscope so the angle of vision is directed toward the uterine horn. Using the lightpost as a guide, rotate the hysteroscope from the 6 o'clock position to inspect the entire cavity.

7. *Patient complains of shoulder pain after sitting up following test.*

   Arranging the examination table in the Trendelenburg position will quickly relieve the shoulder pain. The discomfort is caused by the $CO_2$.

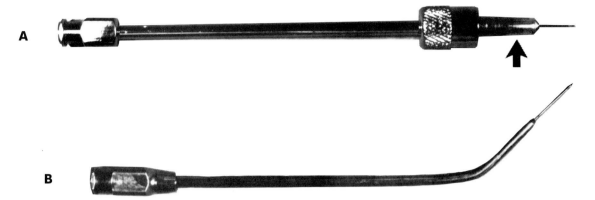

**A**

**B**

FIG. 3-2 Accessories used for injection of local anesthetic include either needle extender (*A*) with attached 25 gauge needle (*arrow*) or (*B*) tonsil needle.

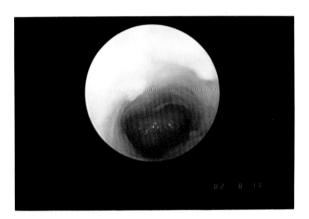

FIG. 3-3 Dark area in background represents uterine fundus.

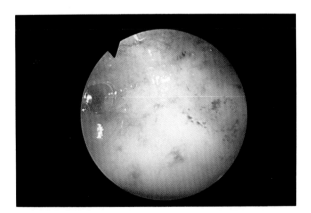

FIG. 3-4 Uterine cavity is seen clearly.

8. *Loss of CO$_2$ at the cervical os.*

   To prevent the loss of gas from the cervical os during the procedure, the tenaculum can be adjusted to narrow the canal or a second tenaculum can be applied. An alternative in rare cases would be to attach a cervical adaptor to the cervix. This cervical adaptor is held in place by negative pressure (Fig. 3-5). A length of tubing is connected to the outflow channel on the operative sheath, and the opposite end is connected to an electronically controlled vacuum device. Inadvertent inclusion of the vaginal mucous membrane must be avoided. For most diagnostic hysteroscopic examinations, CO$_2$ is instilled without the need for the cervical adaptor, provided the cervix is not dilated to more than 5 mm.

9. *The uterus is severely displaced (retroflexion, retroversion).*

   To see a displaced uterus clearly, it may be necessary for the gynecologist to stand during the procedure. These uteri are difficult to explore hysteroscopically.

10. *Bubbles of gas mixed with blood or mucus obscure vision.*

    In most instances waiting for 1 minute, without additional manipulation of the hysteroscope and sheath, will solve this problem.

The most common indications for office hysteroscopy are to locate the cause of abnormal uterine bleeding, to evaluate an abnormal hysterogram, to locate occult IUDs, to classify intrauterine adhesions, and to explore the lower uterine segment to locate the extension of the endometrial adenocarcinoma or defects from previous cesarean deliveries. Hysteroscopy also allows the physician to evaluate the results of therapeutic procedures. Some findings seen in the uterine cavity during office hysteroscopy are shown in Fig. 3-6.

No special postoperative care is needed and infrequent complications indicate a carefully performed procedure.

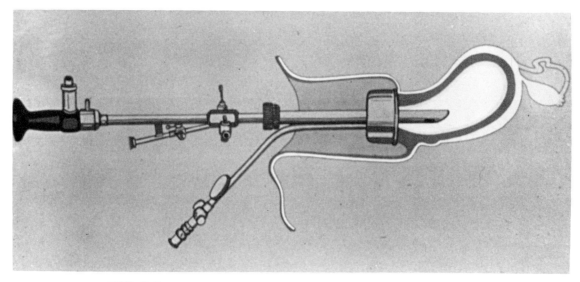

*FIG. 3-5* Cervical suction cups are not used frequently. Drawing shows application of suction cup.

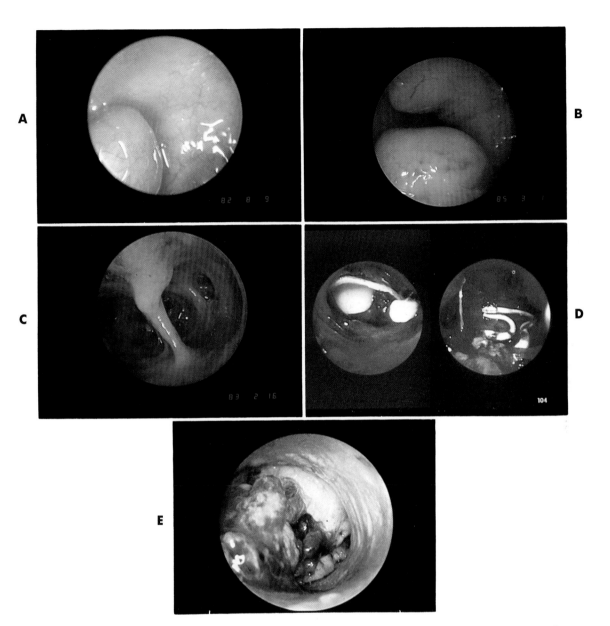

*FIG. 3-6* Some findings seen in uterine cavity during office hysteroscopy. **A**, Endometrial polyp; **B**, Submucous myoma; **C**, Intrauterine adhesions; **D**, Intrauterine device (IUD); **E**, Endometrial adenocarcinoma.

## NORMAL SALINE OR DEXTROSE 5%

A 500 ml plastic bag containing normal saline (NS) or dextrose 5% ($D_5W$) is connected to one of the inflow channels on the sheath with intravenous tubing. They can either be hung on an infusion pole and instilled by gravity flow, or a blood pressure cuff can be placed around the plastic bag and inflated to between 80 to 120 mm Hg to instill the solution. The usual intra-uterine pressures using this system are 40 mm Hg, but pressures of 100 to 110 mm Hg may be required to see the tubal ostia. The outflow of the distention fluid around the instrument is inconvenient and somewhat messy, but it does not hinder performance of the hysteroscopy. Before the hysteroscope and sheath are inserted into the external os, the sheath is flushed to remove air. An alternative method of uterine distention is to manually inject the fluid by attaching a 50 ml syringe to the sheath through an intervening plastic extension tubing.

Since blood and mucus are miscible with NS and $D_5W$, it may be necessary to flush them from the uterine cavity. The pressure of the fluid is sufficient for this task. A simple method for this procedure is to introduce a plastic catheter through the operating channel. The catheter is attached to a 20 ml syringe containing $D_5W$. The opposite out-flow stopcock of the sheath is opened, and flushing performed with the 20 ml–filled syringe. The pressure generated at the tip of the catheter is sufficient to clear the uterine cavity.

Several other methods can be used to deliver low viscosity fluids at a constant pressure, particularly when these solutions are used for operative hysteroscopy and the procedure is lengthy. One of these involves an electrically driven pump designed by Quinones.[14] This apparatus has a manometer and a small compressor that displaces the fluid by pumping air into a glass bottle (Fig. 3-7). Constant pressure that maintains adequate distention of the uterine cavity can be achieved, but one must avoid pumping air directly into the system when there is no more fluid. A built-in filter prevents the reflux of fluid. With another technique, an orthopedic tourniquet is used to maintain a constant intrauterine pressure. The tourniquet is applied to a plastic bag containing low-viscosity fluids. Two bags are used alternatively and changed through Y-tubing connected to the pump.

Diagnostic hysteroscopy can be performed using NS and $D_5W$ as the distention media, but operative procedures are difficult because the solutions mix with blood. These fluids are readily available, relatively inexpensive, easy to infuse, and intravenous intravasation does not cause a problem. A blood pressure cuff (inflated to the proper pressure) around a plastic fluid-filled container can instill the fluid. Normal saline mixes readily with blood and has a refractive index of 1.37 but should not be used if electrosurgery is contemplated. The cavity must be flushed frequently to keep the medium reasonably clear. The solution passes freely through the tubes, enters the peritoneal cavity, and is absorbed readily. If large volumes of sodium-free water enter the circulation, fluid overload can result. Therefore the amount of solution instilled into the uterus must be monitored.[2]

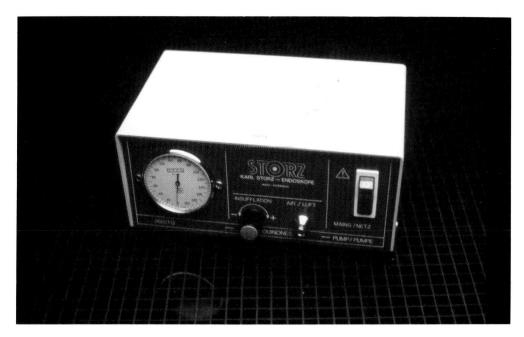

FIG. 3-7 Apparatus developed by Quinones to instill low viscosity fluids during operative hysteroscopy.

**GLYCINE**

Glycine is an aminoacetic acid that has been used by urologists as an irrigating fluid, during transurethral prostatic resection (TUR). Madsen and Madsen[12] measured the effects on serum electrolytes, free hemoglobin, and free ammonia using five types of irrigating fluids during transurethral prostatectomies. Distilled water and 1% urea caused hemolysis and hyperkalemia. None of the fluids (pure distilled water, 1% urea, 3.2% Cytal, 1.5% glycine, or 2.5% dextrose and water) contained enough sodium and hyponatremia was a concern. They calculated that a patient weighing 70 kg, and irrigated with 1000 ml of a 1.5% glycine solution in a 1 hour TUR, absorbed glycine-N at the rate of 0.5 mg/kg/min. There was no direct correlation between the amount of free serum ammonia and clinical symptoms in patients with liver cirrhosis or hepatitis. As an isotonic solution, glycine can eliminate the risk of intravascular hemolysis. It is a nonelectrolytic solution that permits the use of high-frequency current for operative procedures. Glycine appears to be locally nonirritating, and if intravascular intravasation occurs, usually no side effects result. It is transparent, does not interfere with visual acuity during the operation, and is relatively inexpensive, allowing the use of large quantities. Since it lacks electrolytes, the amount of fluid used should be carefully monitored to prevent hypervolemia, hyponatremia, and possible noncardiogenic pulmonary edema. Glycine is metabolized into ammonia in the liver and excreted as urea. It should be used cautiously in patients who have impaired liver or renal function.[15] Glycine is supplied as a 1.5% solution in 3 L containers (Table 3-2).

*Table 3-2* Low Viscosity Fluids (NS, $D_5W$, and Glycine)

| Advantages | Disadvantages |
| --- | --- |
| Several systems available for instillation<br>  Gravity<br>  Blood pressure cuff<br>  Quinones compressor<br>  Orthopedic tourniquet<br>Fluids readily available, inexpensive<br>Refractive index 1.37 | Inconvenient for office hysteroscopy<br>Need constant irrigation to clear debris<br>Saline not recommended with<br>  electrosurgery<br>Large volume needed (liters)<br>Concern for fluid overload |

## HIGH VISCOSITY FLUIDS

Hyskon is a clear, viscid, sterile, nonpyrogenic solution of dextran 70 (32% W/V) in dextrose 10% (W/V). The fluid is electrolyte-free and nonconductive. Dextran is a branched polysaccharide composed of glucose units. Dextran 70 is a fraction of dextran that has an average molecular weight of 70,000. If Hyskon is subjected to temperature variations or stored for long periods of time, it tends to crystallize. The extent of systemic absorption of dextran 70 by the uterine and peritoneal cavities has not been ascertained. The gynecologist must be aware of the potential for anaphylactoid reactions, plasma volume expansion, and prolonged bleeding times. Dextran 70 is also supplied in solutions of saline 6% and water 12%.

The solution is viscous and has excellent optical properties. Blood does not mix with it, so even with intrauterine manipulation and the bleeding that can result, a clear field can be maintained. Electrosurgery can be performed with Hyskon because the solution is nonconductive.[1,8]

A disadvantage of Hyskon is its tendency to adhere to instruments. If it is not washed off with hot water immediately after a procedure, it can damage valves and optical components. The keys to successful use are as follows:

1. To minimize leakage, dilate only enough of the cervix to admit the sheath with a tight fit.
2. Hyskon must be poured slowly down the side of the container to avoid the formation of air bubbles, then aspirated into two or three 50 ml plastic syringes.
3. To eliminate air, the sheath must be filled with the solution before it is inserted into the uterine cavity.
4. If polyethylene tubing is used to connect the filled syringe to the sheath, the tubing is filled before attaching it to the inflow valve on the sheath.
5. To avoid the use of excessive amounts of solution, the assistant instills the fluid as instructed by the surgeon.

Hyskon is usually delivered in small amounts with a handheld syringe. Alternatively, a mechanical device can deliver a preset amount of Hyskon by releasing it at intervals using a foot pedal.[6] The view of the uterine cavity is facilitated because the gynecologist controls the delivery system, and smaller amounts of the distending medium are required. This approach eliminates the need to empty the 100 ml containers of solution into syringes because the original bottle of Hyskon is used as the reservoir. It is attached to the operative sheath by a disposable infusion set, and the $CO_2$ under pressure controls the flow of the liquid medium (Fig. 3-8). The initial uterine distention with this apparatus is performed with a pressure of 300 mm Hg but is limited to the minimal amount required for adequate observations. The pressure required will vary, depending on uterine leakage and should be carefully monitored by the hysteroscopist during the procedure. The foot pedal must be activated only while the infusion bottle is in the inverted or hanging position. This pump uses $CO_2$ from an external high-pressure supply, and a reducing valve is designed to keep the flowrate at safe levels. The drip chamber contains a safety-check ball that is supposed to prevent inadvertent pumping of gas into the uterus of the patient. The disposable plastic infusion set connects the bottle of Hyskon to the gas line in the pump, and a male luer lock fitting connects it to the hysteroscopic sheath. It is important that the operating instructions for this apparatus are read carefully before using.

Large volumes of Hyskon or excessive instillation pressures cause endometrial edema, therefore the contour of the cavity is obscured. The amount of solution used should be monitored and rarely exceed 300 ml; infusion pressures should be no greater than 150 mm Hg. Many investigators consider this fluid to be the medium of choice for operative procedures because the bleeding caused by intrauterine manipulation does not interfere with continued viewing (Table 3-3).

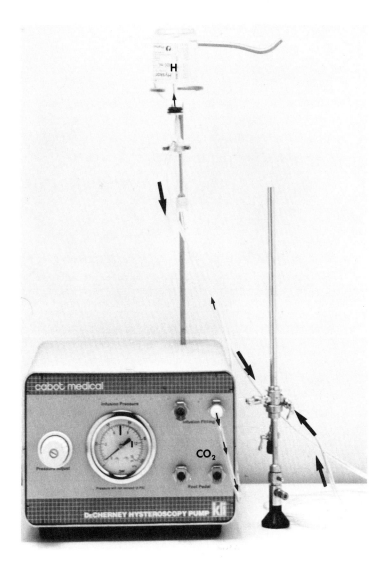

FIG. 3-8 Pump designed to instill Hyskon. Release of foot pedal (not shown) is controlled by surgeon. *Small arrows* indicate direction of flow of $CO_2$ into bottle of Hyskon. *Large arrows* indicate direction of flow of liquid into hysteroscope. (Courtesy of Cabot Medical, Langhorne, Pa.)

*Table 3-3* High Viscosity Fluids (Hyskon)

| Advantages | Disadvantages |
| --- | --- |
| Electrolyte-free, nonconductive | Inconvenient for office hysteroscopy |
| Excellent optical qualities | Potential for anaphylactoid reaction |
| Can be injected with a 50 ml plastic syringe | Adheres to instruments |
| Does not mix well with blood | Need for special insufflator to control instillation |
| Good for therapeutic hysteroscopy | |

## COMPLICATIONS FROM MEDIA
### Gaseous Media

Lindemann and Gallinat[10] reported no changes in electrocardiograms, $P_{CO_2}$, or pH in 40 patients during $CO_2$ hysteroscopy. Hulf et al.[4] studied changes in arterial $P_{CO_2}$ during hysteroscopy when nitrous oxide was used. Arterial $P_{CO_2}$ rose, and in two patients the rise was significant. One of these patients, apparently in good health, developed a profound bradycardia 8 minutes after hysteroscopy was started and required resuscitation. Nitrous oxide is contraindicated as a gaseous medium for uterine distention. Using German shepherd dogs, anesthetized and unanesthetized, the safety of $CO_2$ was studied. $CO_2$ was administered by direct infusion into their femoral veins at a rate of 200 ml/min. Infusion for 5 minutes at this rate caused slight increases in the pulse and deepened breathing. No change in pH or $P_{CO_2}$ was noted. At rates of 400 ml/min, toxic signs appeared and a lethal dose was established at an infusion rate of 1000 ml/min after 60 seconds.[9] Rubin[16] collected the results from over 80,000 $CO_2$ insufflations reported by 380 authors who did not describe any serious side effects. To see the cardiac ventricles, cardiologists have in the past safely insufflated a single dose of 200 ml/min of $CO_2$.

Pulmonary embolism is a theoretic possibility, but the risk is minimal using a controlled gas delivery system. Fatal and nonfatal accidents have occurred with imperfect gas flow monitors. A proper system should limit the flowrate to 100 ml/min, and the intrauterine pressure should not exceed 200 mm Hg. These two aspects monitor one another because the flowrate is reduced automatically as the intrauterine pressure increases. Because of the potentially severe consequences of excessive flowrates, these mechanical insufflators should probably be calibrated every 2 years. It must be emphasized that the insufflator for creating a pneumoperitoneum during laparoscopy should never be used to form the pneumometra in hysteroscopy because the uterus cannot safely tolerate 1 to 2 L/min. Porto[13] cited seven cases of cardiac arrest in which either the $CO_2$ insufflation was not monitored or its flowrate exceeded 350 ml/min. In summary, the settings on the hysteroscopic insufflator will depend on whether the instrument has a constant flow/variable pressure or a constant pressure/variable flow. Although the peritoneal cavity has a large capacity, direct vascular absorption, induced by the $CO_2$, is more likely to occur in the endometrial cavity because of vasodilatation of the many surface endometrial vessels.

## Liquid Media

The ideal fluid used as a hysteroscopic medium is a solution that is isotonic, nonhemolytic, nonconductive, nontoxic if absorbed, and allows clear visibility during an operation. Excretion should be rapid and it should be an osmotic diuretic. Also, the solution should not crystallize on the instruments, and the expansion of plasma and extracellular fluid volume caused by absorption of the fluid should be low and transient.

Potential complications associated with 32% dextran 70 as the distending medium include cardiovascular overload and anaphylactoid reactions.[11] Kaplan and Sabin[5] reported noncardiogenic pulmonary edema with its intravenous use. Zabella et al.[20] described the same complication in two patients while using dextran 70 during operative hysteroscopy. When noncardiogenic pulmonary edema occurs a team approach is essential. A hypervolemic state must be differentiated from transient cardiogenic pulmonary edema. Temporarily decompensated valvular disease or arrhythmias must be ruled out. Anaphylaxis, caused by bronchospasm, is a documented complication that can result in hypoxia. Blood gases should be drawn and a central venous pressure line is needed. Swan-Ganz monitoring of the pulmonary capillary wedge pressure and the intake and output should be carefully monitored, and furosemide (Lasix) administered as indicated. Without hemodynamic measurements of the capillary wedge pressure, definitive conclusions concerning the cause of pulmonary edema are not possible. Clinical dextran is not immunogenic, but sensitivity to dextran or bacterial contamination of commercial dextran has been associated with allergic reactions, including anaphylaxis. Intravascular absorption of 32% dextran 70 can have a direct toxic effect on the pulmonary capillaries, resulting in extravasation and interstitial pulmonary edema.

Intravascular dextran inhibits blood coagulation, which can contribute to postoperative bleeding and hemoptysis. A drop in hemoglobin postoperatively could be caused by hemodilution or hemorrhage. Clotting studies are important for these patients.

The inflow and outflow of liquid media must be carefully measured so that noncardiogenic pulmonary edema can be avoided.[7] The open vascular channels resulting from dissection or endometrial ablation can predispose patients to this problem. The gynecologist must be alert to the early signs of impending fluid overload and institute prompt measures to avoid serious sequelae.

Prolonged hysteroscopic operative procedures (over 60 minutes) require the use of large amounts (over 1000 ml) of solution. Large amounts of glucose and water ($D_5W$) can cause hyponatremia and hyperglycemia. It is important to use solutions with appropriate electrolytes, such as lactated Ringer's, to obviate this potential complication. In any event, the urine output should be properly monitored.

## SUMMARY

The choice of medium depends on the familiarity of the surgeon with that medium, its clarity, ease of instillation, miscibility with blood, complexity of the equipment for its instillation, messiness, and potential side effects. The operative procedure, its duration, and the instruments used are other important aspects to be considered in each case.

## References

1. Amin HK and Neuwirth RS: Operative hysteroscopy utilizing dextran as a distending medium, Clin Obstet Gynecol 26:277, 1983.
2. Carson SA, Hubert GD, Schriock ED, et al.: Hyperglycemia and hyponatremia during operative hysteroscopy with 5% dextrose in water distension medium, Fertil Steril 51:341, 1989.
3. Hamou J: Microcolpohysteroscopy: a new procedure and its original applications in gynecology, J Reprod Med 26:375, 1981.
4. Hulf JA, Corall IM, Strunin L, et al.: Possible hazards of nitrous oxide for hysteroscopy, Br Med J 1:511, 1975.
5. Kaplan AI and Sabin S: Dextran-70: another cause of drug-induced noncardiogenic pulmonary edema, Chest 68:376, 1975.
6. Lavy G, Diamond MP, Shapiro B, et al.: A new device to facilitate intrauterine instillation of Dextran 70 for hysteroscopy, Obstet Gynecol 70:955, 1987.
7. Leake JF, Murphy AA, and Zacur HA: Noncardiogenic pulmonary edema: a complication of operative hysteroscopy, Fertil Steril 48:497, 1987.
8. Levine RU and Neuwirth RS: Evaluation of a method of hysteroscopy with the use of thirty percent dextran, Am J Obstet Gynecol 113:696, 1972.
9. Lindemann HJ: Atlas der Hysteroskopie, Stuttgart, 1980, Gustav Fischer.
10. Lindemann HJ and Gallinat A: Physikalische und physiologische Grundlagen der $CO_2$-Hysteroskopie, Geburtsh Frauenhlk 36:729, 1976.
11. Maddi VI, Wyso EM, and Zinner EN: Dextran anaphylaxis, Angiology 20:243, 1969.
12. Madsen PO and Madsen RE: Clinical and experimental evaluation of different irrigating fluids for transurethral surgery, Invest Urol 3:122, 1965.
13. Porto R: Hystéroscopie. In Encyclopedie, Paris, 1974, Medico-Chirurgie.
14. Quinones RG: Hysteroscopy with a new fluid technique. In Siegler AM and Lindemann HJ, eds: Hysteroscopy: principles and practice, Philadelphia, 1984, JB Lippincott.
15. Roesch RP, Stoelting RK, Lingeman JE, et al.: Ammonia toxicity resulting from glycine absorption during transurethral resection of the prostate, Anesthesiology 58:577, 1983.
16. Rubin IC: Uterotubal insufflation, St. Louis, 1947, The CV Mosby Co.
17. Semm K: Atlas of gynecologic laparoscopy and hysteroscopy, Philadelphia, 1977, WB Saunders (translated by AL Rice).
18. Siegler AM: A comparison of gas and liquid for hysteroscopy, J Reprod Med 15:73, 1975.
19. Siegler AM: Panoramic $CO_2$ hysteroscopy, Clin Obstet Gynecol 26:242, 1983.
20. Zbella EA, Moise J, and Carson SA: Noncardiogenic pulmonary edema secondary to intrauterine instillation of 32% dextran 70, Fertil Steril 43:479, 1985.

# 4 *Contraindications and Complications*

Usually, hysteroscopy is an endoscopic procedure free of complications. Adverse reactions as a result of diagnostic hysteroscopy are fewer than those following therapeutic hysteroscopy. Each stage of the procedure has its own particular hazard, any of which could be made worse by inexperience. Reports of numerous examinations and treatments under hysteroscopic control reveal comparatively few adverse reactions, and these are generally not serious.[16] Faulty techniques and selection of inappropriate patients are the most frequent causes of sequelae.[7]

## CONTRAINDICATIONS
### Absolute Contraindications

When should hysteroscopy not be done? The contraindications are similar to those for hysterosalpingography (Fig. 4-1). After a hysteroscopy, a patient with a history of recent pelvic inflammatory disease or adnexnal tenderness, with or without pelvic mass, can develop salpingitis or peritonitis when either a gaseous or liquid medium was used for distention. Salpingitis is the one absolute contraindication to hysteroscopy. The vaginal area should be free of infection before conducting a hysteroscopic examination. Infection in the lower genital tract can spread to the fallopian tubes by direct extension from the endometrium, by the lymphatic system, or be transported through the blood system.

To avoid the spread of disease, patients who have a cervical malignancy should not have the procedure done. The results of a hysteroscopic examination would not alter the therapy.

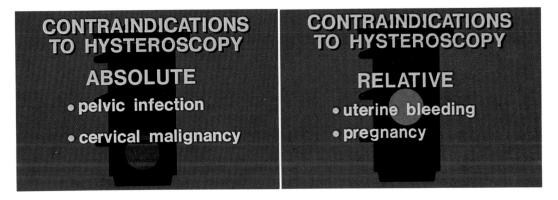

**CONTRAINDICATIONS TO HYSTEROSCOPY**

**ABSOLUTE**
- pelvic infection
- cervical malignancy

**CONTRAINDICATIONS TO HYSTEROSCOPY**

**RELATIVE**
- uterine bleeding
- pregnancy

*FIG. 4-1* Contraindications to hysteroscopy are absolute and relative.

## Relative Contraindications

Scanty or mild uterine bleeding does not prevent adequate observation of the uterine cavity or predispose patients to complications. Regardless of the distending medium used, hysteroscopy cannot be performed satisfactorily if bleeding is excessive. Heavy bleeding should be suppressed so proper interpretation of the endometrial cavity can be made, and vascular intravasation of the distending media will be less likely to occur.

Pregnant women are usually not candidates for hysteroscopy. They should be made aware of the risk of abortion, infection, and bleeding. In select, controlled instances, such as removal of an IUD from a patient who inadvertently becomes pregnant, hysteroscopy can be done without disturbing the pregnancy. Van Lith et al.,[18] using $CO_2$ as the distending medium, described the hysteroscopic findings immediately following postabortal evacuations of 60 patients who were between 14 to 16 weeks' gestation. Although none of the women complained of shoulder pain during or after the test and no serious sequelae were reported, Van Lith et al. urged caution in the use of hysteroscopy to assess the completeness of uterine evacuation. Their study concluded that, although the uterine cavity was usually completely empty, in a few cases when a final suction of the uterine horns had not been done, residual tissue remained and there was obstruction.

Gallinat[5] suggests that there are three indications for hysteroscopy during early pregnancy:

1. To study an IUD in relation to early implantation
2. To perform embryoscopy
3. To evaluate the threatened abortion (the "disturbed" pregnancy)

He observed, before elective abortion, normal changes in the blastocyst implantation from the fifth to the eleventh week of gestation and described the results of $CO_2$ hysteroscopy in 16 pregnant patients who were bleeding.

Salat-Baroux et al.[15] used the hysteroscope to check localized sequelae of uncomplicated cases of elective abortion and detect early complications of spontaneous or induced abortions. The first group studied included 118 patients who had elective abortions before the tenth week of gestation (Table 4-1). The second study included 33 patients, 13 had complications after spontaneous abortion and 20 had complications after elective abortion. The postoperative appearance of the uterine cavity was practically the same when only aspiration was used or when it was combined with curettage. No

*Table 4-1* Elective Abortions—Findings in 118 Patients

| Results | Sequential Hysteroscopic Examinations | | | |
| --- | --- | --- | --- | --- |
| | First Week | Second Week | Third Week | Fourth Week |
| Patients (no.) | 118 | 33 | 17 | 7 |
| Uterus empty | 35 | 6 | 8 | 7 |
| Blood clots | 6 | 0 | 0 | 0 |
| Minimal tissue | 42 | 18 | 5 | 0 |
| Minimal adhesions | 25 | 9 | 4 | 0 |

*Modified from Salat-Baroux J, Hamou JE, Uzan S, et al.: Postabortal hysteroscopy. In Siegler AM and Lindemann HJ, eds: Hysteroscopy: principles and practice, Philadelphia, 1984, JB Lippincott.

untoward effects were noted. When postabortal bleeding occurs, hysteroscopy is a simple method to search for retained placental tissue.

Because few women have such severe cardiovascular disease, hysteroscopy can be accomplished safely using local anesthesia. Indeed a successful hysteroscopic examination, showing a normal uterine cavity, might even allow the patient to avoid a curettage.

## PREVENTION OF COMPLICATIONS
### Infection

To avoid significant problems, the physician should take a careful history and perform a preliminary pelvic examination to identify patients who have occult or overt infections. The hysteroscopic equipment should be disassembled, rinsed and flushed, and disinfected before each examination. The equipment should be rinsed out completely because the solution used to disinfect it can cause irritation of the mucous membranes or peritoneum.[10] Sterilization of the endoscope is not essential.

Disinfection should be done according to the manufacturer's instructions, using a chemical substance that has the capability of killing all microorganisms (gram-positive and gram-negative bacteria, fungi, mycobacteria, and lipophilic and hydrophilic viruses). Corson[1] suggested the following guidelines:

1. Disinfectants such as iodophors and glutaraldehydes can be used.
2. After using this type of disinfectant, rinse with sterile water to prevent possible residual toxic effects of the chemical or detergent.
3. This process should occur after each procedure. Instruments not used immediately should be disinfected and rinsed again before use.
4. Instruments should be thoroughly air dried after cleaning and before storage. Bacteria will multiply in a moist environment.

Because the rate of infection subsequent to hysteroscopy is quite low, any questions regarding the risks associated with liquid media are likely to remain unanswered. If the manufacturer's recommendations concerning disinfecting solutions are followed, infections will not be caused by contaminated instruments.

### Bleeding

Moderate bleeding precludes adequate observation of the cavity, and open vessels predispose the patient to vascular intravasation and possibly embolism. Observations should begin as the sheath and hysteroscope are inserted into the endocervical canal without advancing the instrument, except in a clear field of vision.

### Perforation

A reddened or cloudy view of the uterine cavity may be caused by juxtaposition of the objective lens to the uterine wall, inadequate uterine distention, or a lens with adherent blood or mucus. Additional force can result in uterine perforation and the intestines will quickly come into endoscopic view. Except where endometrial scarring is present and the familiar landmarks cannot be identified, the risk of uterine perforation during hysteroscopic surgery is small. Visual control makes perforation unlikely. Simultaneous laparoscopy reduces the consequences of accidental perforation, and, therefore, it is an important associated procedure in selected patients. Whenever observation is limited because of intrauterine disease, the endoscope should be advanced slowly and gently and always under direct vision.

## COMPLICATIONS
### Trauma

Excessive traction on the tenaculum can cause cervical lacerations. Forceful cervical dilatation can provoke unnecessary bleeding, perforate the lower uterine segment, or create a false passage or tract. Occasionally, during simultaneous laparoscopic examinations, perforations have been seen, but after withdrawal of the hysteroscope, bleeding from the uterine wound is minimal. If the hysteroscope is advanced without panoramic vision or with undue force, perforation becomes a potential hazard. Unless there is concern that there is a bowel injury, laparotomy is seldom required. Simultaneous laparoscopy is indicated in those women in whom the uterine landmarks tend to be obscured, such as severe cases of intrauterine adhesions when the uterine fundus, the cornua, and the uterotubal ostia are not seen. A hysterogram that shows vascular intravasation associated with an abnormal uterine shadow is another indication for a laparoscopically controlled operative hysteroscopy. A uterine perforation can go unnoticed during lysis of severe intrauterine adhesions, and continued manipulation with scissors or biopsy forceps can cause severe intestinal injury.[6] As a precaution, all tissues removed during an operative hysteroscopic examination should be sent for surgical pathologic review.

Lindemann[9] reported only 6 fundal perforations in 5220 hysteroscopic examinations. Parent et al.[12] described 12 cases of uterine perforation; 8 occurred during the hysteroscopic resection of severe intrauterine adhesions, 3 occurred during hysteroscopic examinations of older women, and 1 occurred after a miscarriage, during the search for retained placental tissue. In each instance the patient was observed for a few hours. In the latter case a laparoscopy was done so the uterus could be evacuated without additional trauma. The treatment of the synechiae was postponed because the uterus could no longer be distended and blind resection would have been dangerous. If this accident occurs during a diagnostic examination, using a 5 mm sheath, the consequences are minimal. Obviously the endoscope is withdrawn and the contractions of the myometrium allows the defect to close quickly. If perforation occurs during a therapeutic procedure, one uncontrolled by laparoscopy, the decision to resort to laparoscopy or laparotomy should be left to the judgment of the attending physician. The patient should be informed about the complication and told the consequences are minimal. Nevertheless, the patient should be observed for a few hours for evidence of abdominal bleeding. Uterine perforations occur more often following therapeutic procedures than diagnostic examinations, and more often in the fundus than in the lower uterine segment (Fig. 4-2). A displaced uterus (retroflexion, retroversion), a scarred uterine cavity, or an atrophic uterus are three common conditions predisposing patients to this complication.

Probes inserted into the tubal ostia can create a false passage and perforate the uterotubal junction (Fig. 4-3). Tubal cannulation, in an attempt to overcome proximal tubal obstruction, must be carefully controlled visually, either by concomitant laparoscopy or fluoroscopy.[4,13] A hydrosalpinx can rupture during $CO_2$ insufflation and the gaseous medium can pass into the leaves of the broad ligament (Fig. 4-4).

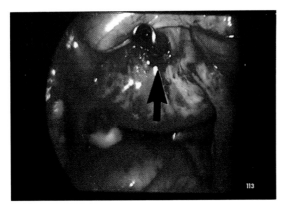

*FIG. 4-2* Operative sheath and hysteroscope have perforated uterine fundus.

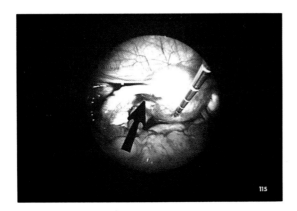

*FIG. 4-3* *Arrow* points to site of small perforation in interstitial tubal segment.

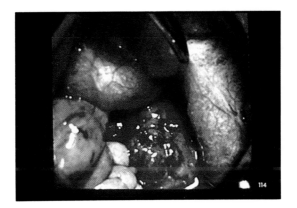

*FIG. 4-4* Fallopian tube ruptured and $CO_2$ entered leaves of broad ligament.

## Electrosurgical Injuries

Currently electrosurgical procedures are being done, mostly without laparoscopic control, to resect submuous myomas and perform endometrial ablation. Since laparoscopy and pneumoperitoneum are not often associated with these procedures, the intestine can be juxtaposed to the uterine serosal surface, and thermal injury can be a potential concern. The width of the myometrium should prevent uterine serosal heating, therefore intestinal injury is avoided. However, a patient who complains of increasing abdominal pain after electrosurgery should be examined promptly for signs of peritonitis. Procrastination can result in severe morbidity or death. Laparotomy, appropriate resection of the injured intestine, drainage, and vigorous antibiotic therapy are necessary.

Hysteroscopic sterilizations had been performed using electrosurgical probes to coagulate the intramural tubal segment. This method fell into disfavor because of serious complications caused by inadvertent thermal injuries to the intestine. The intestine was juxtaposed to the uterine serosal surface, resulting in subsequent peritonitis, and, in a few instances, death.[2] It was apparent that during the hysteroscopic procedure the probes had penetrated the myometrium and perforated the uterus.

## Spread of Carcinoma

No evidence exists to suggest that displaced endometrial fragments result in endometriosis, or that transported endometrial tumor cells metastasize. Several medical centers routinely use hysterosalpingograms (HSG) in the preoperative work-up of patients with endometrial cancer, and no increase in the risk of intraabdominal or distant metastases has been reported.[8,11] In about 50% of the patients with an endometrial carcinoma, contrast medium passed through the fallopian tubes. In the others, the tubes were not patent because the tumor had spread into the myometrium surrounding the intramural segment.[18] In these patients distant metastases were evident earlier, even though the surface spread of the carcinoma appeared limited. During HSG, contrast medium was seen less in the tubes of patients who developed metastases than in those who did not, and the difference was statistically significant.

Although curettage has been the most reliable method for the diagnosis of endometrial carcinoma, some localized lesions can be missed. The use of hysteroscopy to examine patients with endometrial carcinoma has been questioned because cancer can spread through the fallopian tubes into the abdominal cavity. The risk of perforation, hemorrhage, dissemination of cancer cells, and pelvic infection can be avoided if the procedure is done carefully.

Sugimoto[17] performed hysteroscopic examinations in 182 women who had endometrial adenocarcinoma. He found no increased risk for dissemination of cancer cells. Although most tumors were circumscribed, exophytic growths with polypoid, nodular, or papillary processes were often accompanied by necrosis, ulceration, and infection. In another series of 100 patients,[9] hysteroscopy performed using dextran did not cause complications more serious than uterine perforation. No instances of endometritis, salpingitis, or fever were caused by hysteroscopy.

Many small lesions can be detected early; therefore, a prompt diagnosis can lead to suitable treatment with minimal delay. Careful hysteroscopic examination of the endocervix and isthmus can indicate the presence of carcinoma. The extent of the malignancy and the grade of the tumor are the main factors on which to base a therapeutic plan: surgery, radiotherapy, or a combination of both. For prognosis, statistics from several institutions indicate the importance of knowing the extent of the carcinoma.

## Hemorrhage

Slight uterine bleeding a few days subsequent to hysteroscopy can occur, but hemorrhage is unusual. Instances of hemorrhagic shock have not been described. Postoperative bleeding has been reported after resection of submucous myoma, but this complication can be controlled by inserting an intrauterine balloon to tamponade the endometrium. In a report by De-Cherney and Polan,[3] 40 patients were treated for a variety of conditions using the hysteroscopic resectoscope, and nine of these patients experienced postoperative uterine bleeding. In this group, the bleeding was controlled by placing a Foley catheter in the uterine cavity, and the catheter balloon was inflated to provide tamponade. It was left in place for 6 hours, and after removal there were no further hemorrhagic problems. Parent et al.[12] reported that two patients with endometrial adenocarcinoma required transfusions after hysteroscopy because of bleeding. In another instance, a patient needed a hysterectomy after an attempt at hysteroscopic myomectomy.

## Infection

It continues to be quite a surprise to find almost no report of pelvic infection after either diagnostic or therapeutic hysteroscopy. Salat-Baroux et al.[14] noted only seven mild infections in 4000 hysteroscopic examinations, 90% of which were done in an office setting. In addition, cultures of the cervix and the instruments were obtained before and after consecutive use in six patients. All cultures of the instruments and disinfectant before use were negative. After the procedure, cultures were taken from the tip of the hysteroscope and contained the same organisms found in the preoperative cervix. There was no patient-to-patient transmission of bacteria, and no infection occurred in these six patients.

## MORTALITY

The most common cause of death, thus far, has been the media used to distend the uterine cavity during hysteroscopic procedures. Large volumes of $CO_2$, rapidly instilled (>350 ml/min), have resulted in death by pulmonary embolism (Fig. 4-5). Gases such as nitrous oxide and carbon dioxide should never be used to cool sapphire tips mounted on coaxial laser fibers during laser hysteroscopy.[19]

Liquid media have not been implicated in any deaths, but excessive amounts can cause near fatal consequences. The only deaths as the result of overwhelming infections were caused by unsuspected intestinal injuries following therapeutic hysteroscopic procedures, mainly sterilizations.

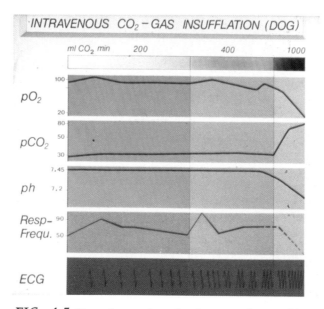

*FIG. 4-5* Experimental study done on dogs subjected to variable amounts and rates of $CO_2$ intravenous insufflation. Significant changes occurred after $CO_2$ at rate of 400 ml/min was injected.

*References*

1. Corson SL: Endoscopy and pelvic infection, Clin Obstet Gynecol 26: 334, 1983.
2. Darabi KF and Richart RM: Collaborative study on hysteroscopic sterilization procedures: preliminary report, Obstet Gynecol 49:48, 1977.
3. DeCherney AH and Polan ML: Hysteroscopic management of intrauterine adhesions and intractable uterine bleeding, Obstet Gynecol 61:392, 1983.
4. DeCherney AH: Anything you can do I can do better . . . or differently! Fertil Steril 48:374, 1987.
5. Gallinat A: Hysteroscopy in early pregnancy. In Siegler AM and Lindemann HJ, eds: Hysteroscopy: principles and practice, Philadelphia, 1984, JB Lippincott.
6. Gentile GP and Siegler AM: Inadvertent intestinal biopsy during laparoscopy and hysteroscopy: a report of two cases, Fertil Steril 36:402, 1981.
7. Graebe RA and DeCherney AH: Avoiding complications in hysteroscopy, Infect Surg 5:146, 1986.
8. Joelsson IS: Hysteroscopy for the delineation of intrauterine extent of endometrial carcinoma. In Siegler AM and Lindemann HJ, eds: Hysteroscopy: principles and practice, Philadelphia, 1984, JB Lippincott.
9. Lindemann HJ: Atlas der Hysteroskopie, Stuttgart, 1980, Gustav Fischer.
10. Loffer FD: Disinfection vs sterilization of gynecologic laparoscopy equipment, J Reprod Med 25:263, 1980.
11. Norman O: Hysterography in cancer of the uterus, Semin Roentgenol 4:244, 1969.
12. Parent B, Guedj H, Barbot J, et al.: Panoramic hysteroscopy, Baltimore, 1987, Williams & Wilkins.
13. Rosh J, Thurmond AS, Ucjida BT, et al.: Selective transcervical fallopian tube catheterization: technique update, Radiology 168:1, 1988.
14. Salat-Baroux J, Hamou JE, Maillard G, et al.: Complications from microhysteroscopy. In Siegler AM and Lindemann HJ, eds: Hysteroscopy: principles and practice, Philadelphia, 1984, JB Lippincott.
15. Salat-Baroux J, Hamou JE, Uzan S, et al.: Postabortal hysteroscopy. In Siegler AM and Lindemann HJ, eds: Hysteroscopy: principles and practice, Philadelphia, 1984, JB Lippincott.
16. Siegler AM: Adverse effects. In Siegler AM and Lindemann HJ, eds: Hysteroscopy: principles and practice, Philadelphia, 1984, JB Lippincott.
17. Sugimoto O, Ushiroyama T, and Fuhuda Y: Diagnostic hysteroscopy for endometrial carcinoma. In Siegler AM and Lindemann HJ, eds: Hysteroscopy: principles and practice, Philadelphia, 1984, JB Lippincott.
18. Van Lith DAF, Schue KV, Beekuizen W, et al.: Carbon dioxide hysteroscopy immediately after second trimester pregnancy termination. In Van Der Pas H, Van Lith DAF, Van Herendael BJ, and Keith LG, eds: Hysteroscopy, Boston, 1983, MTR Press Ltd.
19. Baggish MS, Daniel JF: Death caused by air embolism associated with neodymium: yttrium-aluminum-garnet laser surgery and artificial sapphire tips, Am J Obstet Gynecol 161:877, 1989.

# 5 *Hysteroscopic Metroplasty*

The most common uterine malformations are variations of the double uterus (i.e., septate, bicornuate, didelphys), but many anomalies are never discovered because they are not associated with obstetric or gynecologic difficulties. Ashton et al.[2] reviewed hysterosalpingograms (HSGs) obtained to evaluate tubal closures of normal multiparous women after transcervical sterilization, using methylcyanoacrylate with the female contraceptive device FEMCEPT. Of the 840 HSGs studied, 16 congenital uterine anomalies were identified, an incidence of 1.9%. They were bicornuate/septate types; all of the women had normal reproductive histories. The criterion for identifying this anomaly was the appearance of a midline, triangular-shaped symmetric filling defect extending toward the internal os for 50% or more of the vertical uterine length.

## EMBRYOLOGY

In the absence of the müllerian inhibiting factor (MIF) produced by the functioning testis, the müllerian ducts normally appear in the second month of fetal life. The uterus is of paramesonephric origin and is derived from the fusion of caudal parts of the hollow müllerian ducts, while the upper or superior portions become the fallopian tubes. The greater part of each mesonephric duct atrophies in the female, beginning early in the third month. Those portions that persist become ducts of the epoophoron. Gartner's ducts remain as vestigial structures at any growth level between the epoophoron and the hymen. Since the urinary and reproductive tracts are related embryologically, a fundamental study of women with malformed reproductive organs is incomplete unless investigation includes radiologic investigation of the urinary tract. Rock and Jones[25] found congenital absence of one kidney in 9% of patients with genital anomalies.

Uterine anomalies represent a heterogeneous group of congenital malformations that result from arrested development, abnormal formations, or incomplete fusion of müllerian ducts. A classification proposed by the American Fertility Society seems flexible enough to fit most possibilities (Fig. 5-1).[1]

# THE AMERICAN FERTILITY SOCIETY CLASSIFICATION OF MULLERIAN ANOMALIES

Patient's Name _____ Date _____ Chart # _____

Age _____ G _____ P _____ Sp Ab _____ VTP _____ Ectopic _____ Infertile Yes _____ No _____

Other Significant History ( i.e. surgery, infection, etc. ) _____

_____

HSG _____ Sonography _____ Photography _____ Laparoscopy _____ Laparotomy _____

## EXAMPLES

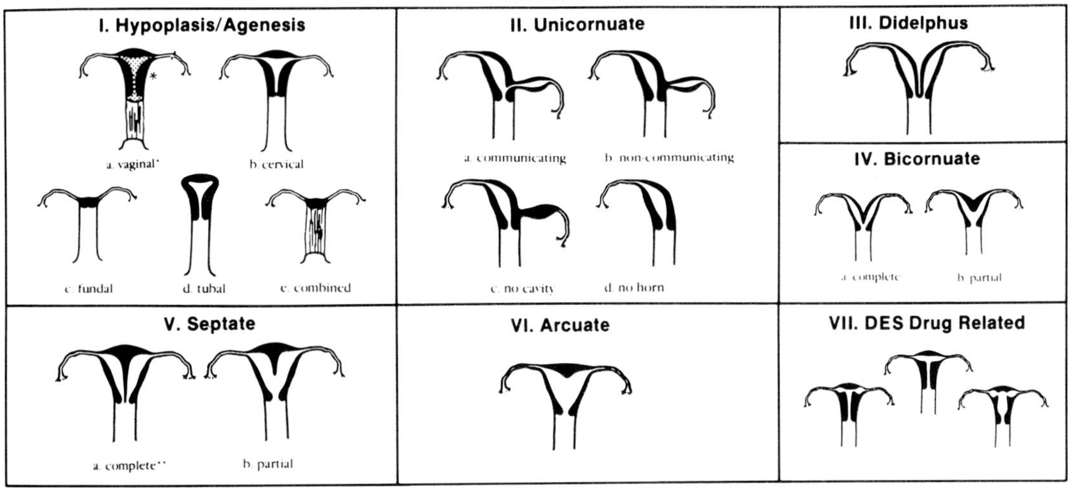

| I. Hypoplasis/Agenesis | II. Unicornuate | III. Didelphus |
|---|---|---|
| a. vaginal*  b. cervical  c. fundal  d. tubal  e. combined | a. communicating  b. non-communicating  c. no cavity  d. no horn | |
| | | IV. Bicornuate |
| | | a. complete  b. partial |

| V. Septate | VI. Arcuate | VII. DES Drug Related |
|---|---|---|
| a. complete**  b. partial | | |

* Uterus may be normal or take a variety of abnormal forms.
** May have two distinct cervices

**Type of Anomaly**

Class I  _____  Class V  _____
Class II  _____  Class VI  _____
Class III  _____  Class VII  _____
Class IV  _____

**Treatment (Surgical Procedures):**  _____

_____

_____

**Prognosis for Conception & Subsequent Viable Infant***

_____ Excellent  ( > 75% )

_____ Good  ( 50-75% )

_____ Fair  ( 25%-50% )

_____ Poor  ( < 25% )

*Based upon physician's judgment.

**Recommended Followup Treatment:**  _____

_____

_____

Property of
The American Fertility Society

**Additional Findings:** _____

_____

_____

Vagina: _____
Cervix: _____

Tubes: Right _____ Left _____
Kidneys: Right _____ Left _____

**DRAWING**

L                                                      R

For additional supply write to:
The American Fertility Society
2140 11th Avenue, South
Suite 200
Birmingham, Alabama 35205

*FIG. 5-1* Classification of uterine anomalies proposed by American Fertility Society. From The American Fertility Society: The American Fertility Society classifications of adnexal adhesions, distal tubal occlusion, tubal occlusion secondary to tubal ligation, tubal pregnancies, Müllerian anomalies and intrauterine adhesions. Fertil Steril 49:944, 1988. Reproduced with permission of the publisher, The American Fertility Society.

## DIAGNOSIS

The physician, by completing prompt and accurate diagnoses, can inform the patient about the reproductive implications and obstetric consequences of uterine anomalies. Some diagnoses can be made by a pelvic examination or by palpation of a heart-shaped fundus during pregnancy and others by means of ultrasonography (US), hysterography, curettage, and pelvic endoscopy (hysteroscopy and laparoscopy) (Fig. 5-2). Although the HSG is an excellent screening test used to detect uterine anomalies, it is limited to the delineation of the uterine cavity. It cannot show the uterine serosal surface. The presence or absence of noncommunicating uterine horns and segmental aplasia or hypoplasia can be disclosed by laparoscopy.[4] Additionally, the physician can discover associated pelvic abnormalities such as endometriosis or periadnexal adhesions.

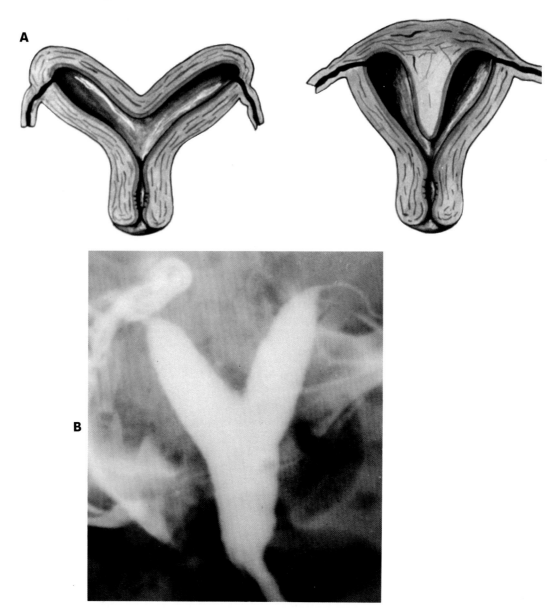

*FIG. 5-2* **A**, Schematic representation showing bicornuate and septate uteri. **B**, HSG reveals V-shaped fundal defect caused by uterine septum.

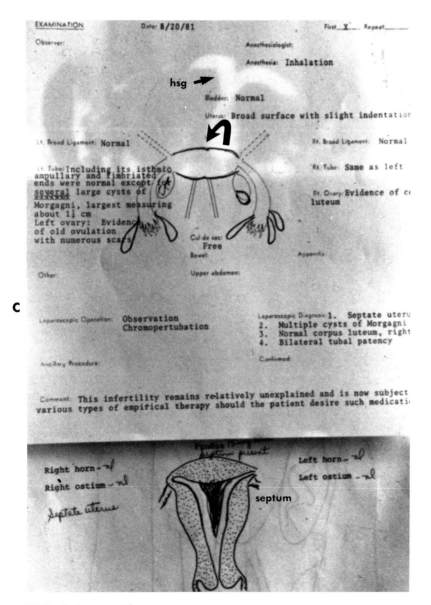

*FIG. 5-2, cont'd* C, Composite of septum seen at hysteroscopy. Laparoscopic findings of normal uterine serosal surface (*curved arrow*) and HSG revealing widely separated uterine horns (*straight arrow*).

## THE SEPTATE UTERUS

Only the septate uterus is amenable to hysteroscopic metroplasty. These uteri are either completely or partially divided by a longitudinal septum. The complete septum may have a small opening that connects to the opposite cavity. Pregnancy wastage indicates the need for a metroplasty, but some procedures have been done to alleviate long-standing infertility when no other reason for the infertility could be ascertained. When viewing the HSG, a uterine septum should be suspected if the fundal angle, caused by separation of the uterine horns, is less than 90%. Although this separation tends to remain constant as the cervix is manipulated with a tenaculum during fluoroscopic control, this observation cannot definitely differentiate the septate uterus from the bicornuate type.[27] The length and width of the fundal septum cause different shadows on the hysterogram, and, if the septum is complete, two separate, usually symmetrical cavities are formed. A cannula inserted beyond the internal os can result in inadequate observation of one cavity and an erroneous diagnosis of a unicornuate uterus.

Pelvic ultrasound helps evaluate uterine anomalies, especially in patients who have obstructive anomalies that can cause a hematocolpos, hematometra, or a hematosalpinx. Recent publications show that US[14] and magnetic resonance imaging (MRI)[21] are good diagnostic methods for ascertaining the type of uterine malformation. Using these techniques it has become possible to locate the uterine serosal surface and to measure the depth of the fundal indentation. To obtain an optimal view of the endometrial cavity, both procedures are performed in the second half of the menstrual cycle since the endometrium is thicker and easily identified. Scans allowing the physician to see the endometrium and serosal uterine surfaces simultaneously must be obtained from as close as possible to the plane containing the ostia and internal os. The use of US has been proposed not only to differentiate between bicornuate and septate uteri but also to monitor hysteroscopic surgery. US is performed with transabdominal or vaginal sectorial probes. The transabdominal study requires a full bladder, and sometimes a liquid medium is needed to distend the uterine cavity. The US examination of the uterus should provide information about: (1) its anterior-posterior and transverse diameters; (2) the contour of the serosal surface; (3) the endometrial lining; and (4) the length of the septum dividing the uterine cavity (Fig. 5-3). Perino et al.[24] studied 40 women with suspected septate uteri. This condition was subsequently confirmed by laparoscopy in 95% of them. An increased transverse diameter was noted in 80% of the patients, and a double cavity was seen in 45% of them. The identification of a hyperechogenic median septum was possible only nine times (22.5%).

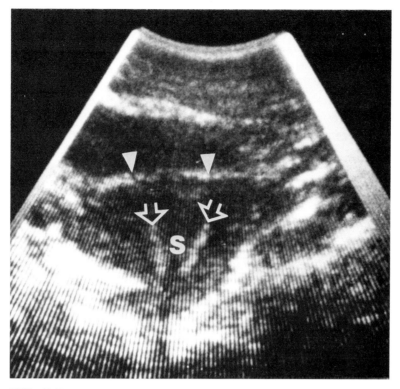

*FIG. 5-3* Ultrasonography clearly demonstrates intact uterine serosal surface (*arrowheads*) and two cavities caused by a septum (*open arrows*).

The differential diagnosis includes the arcuate uterus, which is a minor uterine malformation caused by failure of complete fusion of müllerian ducts. The diagnosis can be presumed from the hysterogram if a line drawn from one cornu to the other and another perpendicular to it and extending to the depth of the concavity measures between 1 and 1.5 cm; if its angle is more than 100%; if the uterine horns appear symmetrical; and if the contour is that of a saddle-shaped fundus (Fig. 5-4). The arcuate uterus is considered a normal variant and is not associated with infertility or obstetrical difficulties. The external contour of the arcuate uterus is normal and can be corroborated by ultrasound. During hysteroscopic examination the fundal protrusion is seen as smooth and broad with no well-defined uterine division. Asymmetric uterine horns or an irregular depression suggest a fundal myoma. A hysteroscopic examination of a submucous fundal myoma might reveal its sessile base and characteristic surface vasculature. The uterine horns and uterotubal ostia are not located in a symmetrical position. The small uterine septum (a subseptate uterus) has a more or less V-shaped trough and the fundal depression exceeds 1.5 cm. The septum appears short and bisects only the fundus.

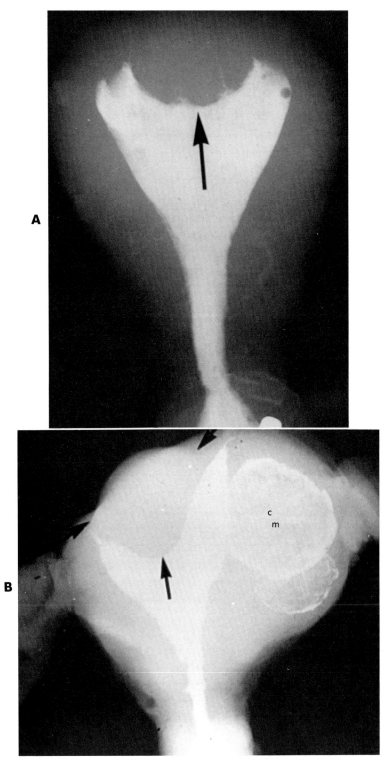

*FIG. 5-4* **A,** Arcuate fundus (*arrow*) seen on HSG. **B,** Specimen shows fundal depression caused by myoma (*arrows*). Calcified myomas (*cm*) are seen on left.

The unique characteristics of the uterus affected by prenatal exposure to diethylstilbestrol (DES) seen on the HSG are a small, hypoplastic endometrial cavity, concavities beneath the cornua that give the appearance of uterotubal constrictions, a T-shaped uterine configuration, and cervical widening (Fig. 5-5). Almost one half of the females who were exposed to DES in utero show some or all of these abnormalities.[20] These radiologic changes can be explained by hysteroscopic examination of the structural alterations within the myometrium that resemble submucous myomas. This appearance is caused by muscular hypertrophy and maldevelopment.

With the hysteroscope, the gynecologist can see the uterine cavity directly and correct certain anomalies such as the septate uterus. The proliferative phase is best for endoscopic study (Fig. 5-6, *A*). The hysteroscopic examination is needed to confirm the fundal abnormality seen radiographically. Laparoscopy is the most accurate method for differentiating between the bicornuate and septate uterus (Fig. 5-6, *B*). The septate uterus, in most cases, has a normal serosal surface, often with a slight increase in transverse diameter. In some patients it may be possible to see a whitish triangle of tissue in the median area that indicates the fundal origin of the septum. Laparoscopy may be required for some patients to monitor hysteroscopic metroplasty.

## SELECTION OF PATIENTS

Data suggest that patients with a septate uterus are twice as likely to abort as those with a bicornuate uterus, and the incidence of abortion is higher for women who have a complete septum. There is little evidence that they are less likely to conceive than patients who have normal uteri. Buttram and Gibbons[3] reported 88% of pregnancies in patients who had a complete septate uterus and 70% in those with a partial septum ended in fetal loss. In 52 patients with uterine septa, Perino et al.[24] found 37 patients who had a previous pregnancy that ended in spontaneous abortion. March and Israel[22] analyzed the outcome of 240 pregnancies in 57 women before metroplasty and noted that 212 pregnancies resulted in miscarriage during the first or second trimester, 7 pregnancies went to term, 21 pregnancies resulted in premature delivery, and only 12 of the premature infants survived.

When the uterus has a septum, the latter is supplied indirectly by uterine vessels, and the increased abortion rate can be explained by the decreased functional intracavitary volume. The endometrium covering the septum, studied in 12 cases, was compared with specimens obtained from biopsies of other areas in the uterine cavity. No significant differences were noted.[3] The ideal patient for metroplasty should have had at least two abortions with a classic history of pain and delivered an identifiable fetus late in the first trimester. Other causes of a miscarriage should be ruled out by a properly timed endometrial biopsy, cervical culture for chlamydia, appropriate endocrinologic tests, karyotyping of both partners, and an intravenous pyelogram.

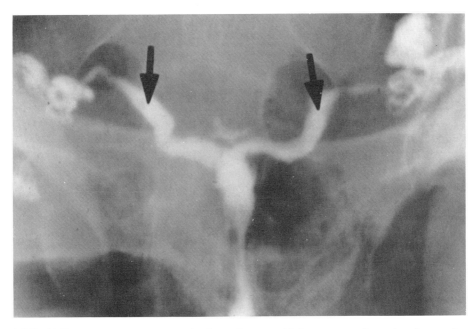

*FIG.* 5-5 Malformed uterine shadow shows widely separated uterine horns (*arrows*) resulting from DES exposure in utero.

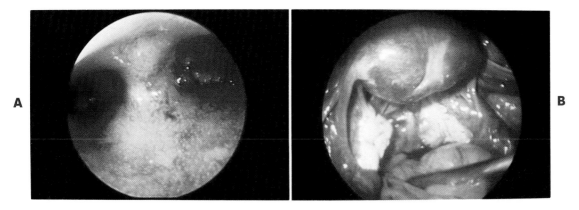

*FIG.* 5-6 **A,** Uterine septum separates two uterine horns and extends about 2 cm into uterine cavity. **B,** Laparoscopic view of intact, slightly indented, uterine serosal surface.

## HYSTEROSCOPIC METROPLASTY

This technique was proposed originally by Edström in 1974,[12] but the method was used infrequently until improvements in illumination, distension media, and accessory instruments were developed. The hysteroscopic examination should afford a good panoramic view of both uterine horns, the uterotubal ostia and the base of the septum before the dissection is begun. The objective of the procedure is to create a uniform, symmetrical cavity and to convert its Y-shape into an equilateral triangle (Fig. 5-7). In their series, DeCherney et al.[11] discovered that the lengths of the septa varied from 1 to 4 cm, and the patients were considered inoperable if the base of the septum was more than 1 cm wide. Technical difficulties can be caused by a wide septum, but this abnormality can be corrected with miniature, semirigid scissors or laser vaporization.

Most hysteroscopic metroplasties have been done in the ambulatory operative suite under general anesthesia. Endotracheal intubation is used if laparoscopy is employed to monitor the procedure. The procedures should require no more than 30 to 40 minutes. Media used to distend the uterine cavity include dextran 70 (Hyskon), $CO_2$,[7] $D_5W$, NS,[10] and glycine. Glycine is not viscous, does not conduct electricity, and causes no sequelae if vascular intravasation occurs. Although either liquid or gaseous media can distend the uterine cavity, liquid media are preferred for therapeutic hysteroscopic procedures. Saline cools the uterine wall during laser vaporization or photocoagulation of the septum and does not bubble like dextran 70 when laser energy is used.

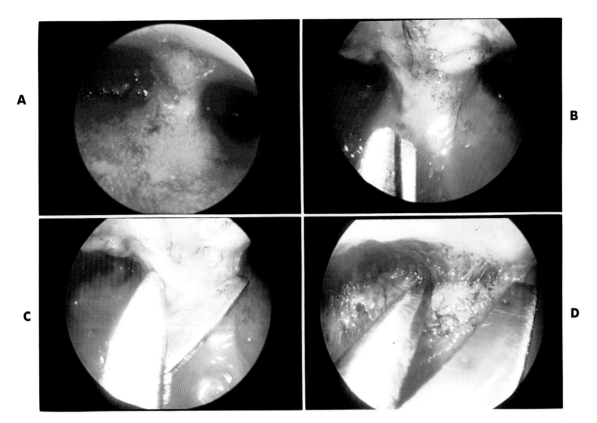

FIG. 5-7 A, Broad uterine septum seen at hysteroscopy. B, Unopened blades of semirigid scissors are noted. C, Opened blades surround septum. D, Septum almost completely incised.

## Hysteroscopic Instruments

Operative instruments include a wire loop urologic resectoscope (8 mm diameter) and flexible, semirigid or rigid scissors of about 7 Fr used through a 21 Fr sheath. The external diameters of the operative sheaths range from 7 to 9 mm. An alternative technique involves dividing the septum by inserting scissors into the uterine cavity along the cervical canal parallel to the hysteroscope. Most accessory instruments are passed through an operative sheath because it is difficult to maneuver two separate instruments along the cervical canal. Septal transection rather than resection is the procedure of choice. Initially the uterine cavity is scanned to evaluate the length and width of the septum and then it is divided until the uterotubal ostia can be seen simultaneously. The incomplete, thin septum is easy to transect. The complete, broad septum is more difficult because septal tissues float in the cavity during the operation and vision becomes obscured. A probe is inserted into one cavity of the cervical septum and a hole is made in it at the level of the internal os. The distending medium tends to leak out of the opposite uterine cavity, but the problem can be circumvented by the insertion of a balloon catheter into one uterine horn to prevent the escape of the medium, or one external os can be occluded with a tenaculum (Fig. 5-8). The cervical partition is not removed because it is believed that after its removal the patient is likely to develop an incompetent os.[18,19] Rock et al.[26] used the resectoscope for lysis of a complete uterine septum leaving the cervical septum intact.

Various instruments have been used for septal incision. March and Israel,[22] Perino et al.,[23] Daly et al.,[8] and Valle and Sciarra[28] use miniature scissors for the incision. This semirigid instrument is small enough to pass through the operating sheath. The blades can be opened to a width that makes it possible to cut even thick septa. Some gynecologists prefer the urologic resectoscope. When electrosurgery is used, 30 W of cutting current are applied in a nonelectrolytic distending medium. Hamou et al.[17] employ an electric knife that is passed through the operating sheath. Electrosurgical cutting current is used with a monopolar electrode. Daniell[10] used the KTP/532 or argon laser, and Goldrath et al.[16] employed the Nd:YAG. The laser septal transection is done with optical fibers 0.6 mm in diameter (Fig. 5-9). The KTP/532 and argon lasers cut by vaporization. There is minimal bleeding and penetration is no more than 1 to 2 mm. When using either of these lasers, eye protection is essential since the backscatter from the beam can damage the surgeon's eye. Filters must be used in the ocular of the hysteroscope, or the procedure done using a video monitor to observe the procedure.

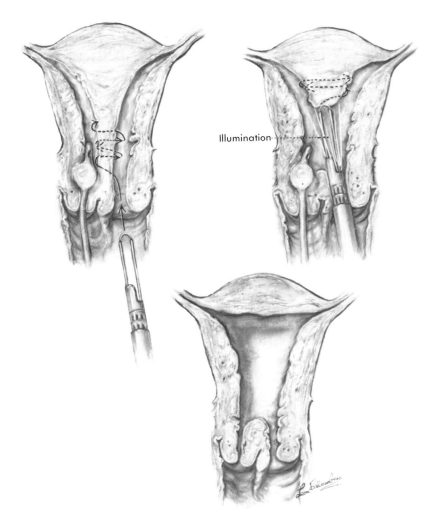

Illumination

*FIG. 5-8* Lysis of complete septum leaving cervical septum intact. (Courtesy of John Rock, MD.)

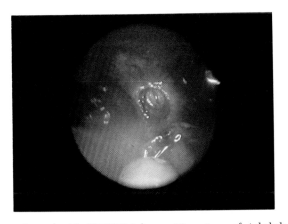

*FIG. 5-9* Septum is cut with KTP/532 laser. (Courtesy of Adolph Gallinat, MD.)

The most delicate part of the procedure is deciding when the transection is complete. One final step is to clearly observe both tubal orifices simultaneously, under panoramic vision. Another is to watch for the presence of small vessels that bleed and pulsate, indicating myometrial bleeding. US can be used for a precise preoperative measurement of the septum and for monitoring the subsequent operation to avoid involvement of the myometrium. Pitressin can be injected into the cervical tissue or even translaparoscopically inserted into the uterine fundus to minimize bleeding. The uterine cavity can be washed by attaching an aspiration catheter to clear the operative field.

The most common intraoperative complication is uterine perforation, but no intestinal injuries have been reported. If the uterus is perforated during the procedure the patient should be informed because it is possible that a subsequent labor could result in a ruptured uterus.

### Preoperative and Postoperative Adjunctive Therapy

Although danazol and GnRh analogs have been prescribed for periods of 30 days to 3 months to initiate endometrial atrophy, reduce vascularization, and halt intraoperative bleeding, the administration of such medication would seem counterproductive. Intraoperative bleeding should not be a problem, if the septum alone was transected, and epithelial regeneration can be promoted by endogenous estrogens. Indeed, postoperative hormone therapy has been suggested for 1 to 2 months in the form of conjugated estrogens and medroxyprogesterone.

Placement of an intrauterine device (IUD) has been advocated to reduce the potential formation of intrauterine adhesions. Fortunately, synechiae are an uncommon postoperative finding. Most physicians do not prescribe the use of antibiotic prophylaxis. Because of increased experience and generally good results, most perioperative medications are no longer needed following hysteroscopic metroplasty.

## THE FOLLOW-UP EXAMINATION

About 2 months postoperatively, either a HSG or hysteroscopic examination is advisable. The hysteroscopic examination may reveal a white scar along the site of the previous septum (Fig. 5-10). The HSG can show a uterine cavity that appears slightly reduced in size, with an arched or arcuate type of fundus and two small "dog-eared" cornua. This does not indicate a poor result, since gestational capacity of the uterine cavity has been improved. Postoperative evaluations indicate that over 90% of septa have been removed successfully. Rock and Jones[25] noted a one-third reduction in the size of the uterine cavity after wedge resection metroplasty done during laparotomy but found no postoperative reduction of successful pregnancies. Following a hysteroscopic metroplasty there can be an increase in total uterine volume. Sometimes the uterine cavity appears cylindrical rather than triangular, but this configuration does not have a deleterious effect on the obstetric outcome.

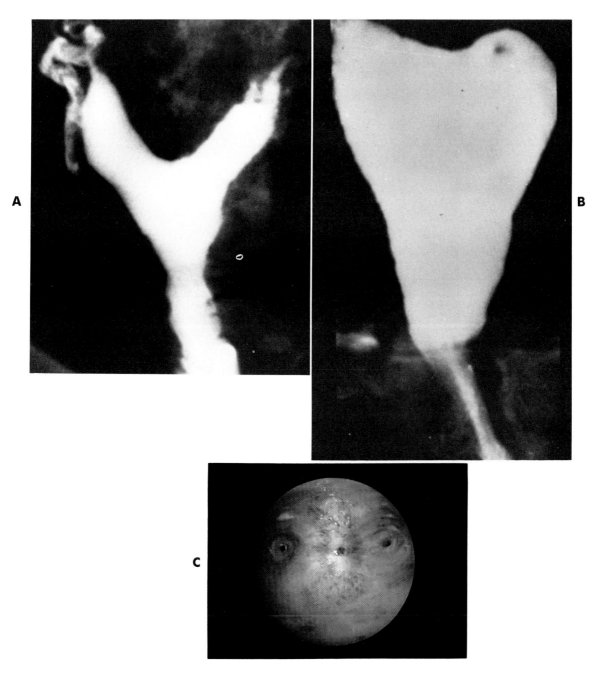

*FIG. 5-10* **A**, Preoperative HSG shows fundal defect caused by uterine septum. **B,** Postoperative HSG reveals normal uterine shadow. **C,** Hysteroscopic view 1 month after surgery discloses symmetrical uterine cavity with central white scar at site of previous septum.

## RESULTS

The criteria for evaluating results include:
1. The feasibility (operability) rate
2. The morphology (configuration) of the postoperative uterine cavity
3. The percentage of term pregnancies

Chervenak and Neuwirth[6] in 1981 reported two cases of hysteroscopic metroplasty that subsequently resulted in term pregnancies. In 1983 Daly et al.[9] successfully incised septa in 25 patients. Preoperatively, there were 40 pregnancies in 17 of these women, and only 1 pregnancy went to term. Postoperatively, there were 6 pregnancies that went to term, 1 preterm delivery at 33 weeks, and 1 immature delivery at 21 weeks. Three patients experienced bleeding from the septum during the operative procedure. The bleeding obscured the operative field before the incision was completed, and 2 months later these patients underwent a repeat hysteroscopic metroplasty. In 1986 DeCherney et al.[11] attempted 103 hysteroscopic resections, 72 were completed successfully. Thirty-one patients were considered inoperable, because the base of the septum was more than 1 cm in width, a feasibility rate of 69%. Of the 72 completed procedures, 58 (80.5%) resulted in successful deliveries. March and Israel[22] described 91 hysteroscopic resections performed in a 4-year period. Of these, 79 were performed because of one or more previous spontaneous abortions. The pretreatment reproductive wastage was 95%. Of the women who became pregnant after therapy, 87% of the pregnancies resulted in a live birth or had gone beyond 20 weeks of gestation. Successful outcomes such as these equal or exceed those achieved by transabdominal metroplasty (Table 5-1). Fayez[13] compared two groups of patients. A laparotomy procedure, known as Tompkins metroplasty, was performed on one group and on the other group, hysteroscopic metroplasty. In the laparotomy series, the pregnancy rate was 71.4%. Of these women, 80% delivered by cesarean section, and the other 20% had spontaneous abortions. Following a hysteroscopic metroplasty, 84% of the patients became pregnant, 78% of them term pregnancies delivered vaginally, but 13% of the deliveries were premature, and 9% experienced recurrent spontaneous abortions.

The main advantages of hysteroscopic metroplasty are as follows:
1. The operation may be performed on an outpatient basis
2. No abdominal or uterine scar results
3. Postoperative morbidity is minimal
4. No reduction in the volume of the uterine cavity results
5. Pregnancy may be attempted after either the postoperative hysteroscopy or hysterogram are normal
6. Vaginal delivery is typical

Table 5-1 Hysteroscopic Metroplasty

| Author | Cases (No.) | Medium Used | Technique | IUD in Place | Estrogen/ progestogen Treatment | Pregnancy | | | |
|---|---|---|---|---|---|---|---|---|---|
| | | | | | | Term | Spontaneous Abortion | Premature | Undelivered |
| Edström[12] | 2 | Hyskon | Rigid biopsy forceps | Yes | No | 0 | 0 | 1 (19 wks) | 0 |
| Chervenak/Neuwirth[6] | 2 | Hyskon | Scissors adjacent hysteroscope | Yes | Yes | 1 | 0 | 0 | 0 |
| Daly et al.[9] | 25 | Hyskon | Semirigid scissors | No | Yes | 7 | 1 | 0 | 2 |
| DeCherney et al.[11] | 72 | Hyskon | Resectoscope | No | No | 58 | 4 | 0 | 0 |
| Corson/Batzer[7] | 18 | $CO_2$/Hyskon | Rigid scissors/ resectoscope | No | No | 10 | 2 | 1 | 2 |
| Fayez[13] | 19 | Hyskon | Rigid scissors | Yes (foley) | No | 14 | 0 | 0 | 0 |
| March/Israel[22] | 91 | Hyskon | Flexible scissors | Yes | Yes | 44 | 7 | 4 | 7 |
| Valle/Sciarra[28] | 59 | Hyskon/$D_5$W | Flexible/rigid/ semirigid scissors | No | Yes | 44 | 5 | 2 | 0 |
| Daniell et al.[10] | 18 | Saline | Laser KTP/argon | No | Yes | NA | 0 | NA | 10 |
| Perino et al.[24] | 61 | $CO_2$/glycine | Semirigid scissors/ resectoscope | No | No | 38 | 4 | 0 | 0 |
| TOTALS | 367 | | | | | 216 | 23 | 8 | 21 |

The outcome is unknown for 99 pregnancies.
NA, Not available.

Hysteroscopic metroplasty is the treatment of choice for management of the uterine septum in the patient who has a reproductive history of repeated fetal loss during the first or second trimester. These results compare favorably with those of metroplasty performed using laparotomy.[5] Uterine septa should probably be removed from patients who have unexplained infertility; then methods such as in vitro fertilization, embryo transfer, or gamete intrafallopian tube transfer (GIFT) might have more successful results. Genell and Sjovall[15] wrote that 13 of 58 women who underwent a Strassmann metroplasty were experiencing primary infertility. In a series of 91 hysteroscopic metroplasties done by March and Israel,[22] 10 women included were experiencing primary infertility, and in the study done by Perino et al.,[24] of 52 operations performed, 15 (28%) involved infertility.

## References

1. American Fertility Society: The American Fertility Society classifications of adnexal adhesions, distal tubal occlusion, tubal occlusion secondary to tubal ligation, tubal pregnancies, müllerian anomalies and intrauterine adhesions, Fertil Steril 49:944, 1988.
2. Ashton D, Amin HK, Richart RM, et al.: The incidence of asymptomatic uterine anomalies in women undergoing transcervical tubal sterilization, Obstet Gynecol 72:28, 1988.
3. Buttram VC and Gibbons WB: Müllerian anomalies: a proposed classification (an analysis of 144 cases), Fertil Steril 32:40, 1979.
4. Buttram VC and Reiter RC: Uterine anomalies. In Buttram VC and Reiter RC, eds: Surgical treatment of the infertile female, Baltimore, 1985, Williams & Wilkins.
5. Capraro VJ, Chuang JT, and Randall CL: Improved fetal salvage after metroplasty, Obstet Gynecol 31:97, 1968.
6. Chervenak FA and Neuwirth RS: Hysteroscopic resection of the uterine septum, Am J Obstet Gynecol 141:351, 1981.
7. Corson S and Batzer FR: $CO_2$ uterine distension for hysteroscopic septate incision, J Reprod Med 31:713, 1986.
8. Daly DC, Tohan N, Walters C, Riddick DH, et al.: Hysteroscopic resection of the uterine septum in the presence of a septate cervix, Fertil Steril 39:560, 1983.
9. Daly DC, Walters CA, Soto-Albors CE, Riddick DH, et al.: Hysteroscopic metroplasty: surgical technique and obstetrical outcome, Fertil Steril 39:623, 1983.
10. Daniell JF, Osher S, and Miller W: Hysteroscopic resection of uterine septi with visible light laser energy, Colpos Gynecol Laser Surg 3:217, 1987.
11. DeCherney AH, Russell JB, Graebe RA, and Polan ML: Resectoscopic management of müllerian fusion defects, Fertil Steril 45:726, 1986.
12. Edström K: Intrauterine surgical procedures during hysteroscopy, Endoscopy 6:175, 1974.
13. Fayez JA: Comparison between abdominal and hysteroscopic metroplasty, Obstet Gynecol 68:399, 1986.
14. Fedele L, Ferrazi E, Dorta M, et al.: Ultrasonography in the differential diagnosis of "double" uteri, Fertil Steril 50:361, 1988.
15. Genell S and Sjovall A: The Strassmann operations: results obtained in 58 cases, Acta Obstet Gynecol Scand 38:477, 1959.
16. Goldrath MH, Fuller TA, and Segal S: Laser photovaporization of endometrium for the treatment of menorrhagia, Am J Obstet Gynecol 140:14, 1981.
17. Hamou JE, Mencaglia L, and Perino A: L'Électroresection en hystéroscopie et microcolpohystéroscopie des fibromes sous-muqueux. In Cittidini E, Scarselli G, Mencaglia L, Perino A, eds: Isteroscopia Operativa e Laser Chirurgia in Ginecologia, Rome, 1988, CIC Edizioni Internationali.
18. Jones HW Jr: Reproductive impairment and the malformed uterus, Fertil Steril 36:137, 1981.

19. Jones HW Jr and Jones GES: Double uterus as an etiological factor of repeated abortion: indication for surgical repair, Am J Obstet Gynecol 65:325, 1976.
20. Kaufman RH, Adam E, Noller K, et al.: Upper genital tract changes and infertility in diethylstilbestrol-exposed women, Am J Obstet Gynecol 154:1312, 1986.
21. Letterie GS, Wilson J, and Miyazawa K: Magnetic resonance imaging of müllerian tract abnormalities, Fertil Steril 50:365, 1988.
22. March CM and Israel R: Hysteroscopic management of recurrent abortion caused by septate uterus, Am J Obstet Gynecol 156:834, 1987.
23. Perino A, Mencaglia L, Hamou J, et al.: Hysteroscopy for metroplasty of uterine septa: a report of 24 cases, Fertil Steril 48:321, 1987.
24. Perino A, Catinella E, Comparetto G, et al.: Hysteroscopic metroplasty: the role of ultrasound in the diagnosis and monitoring of patients with uterine septa, Acta Eur Fertil 18:349, 1987.
25. Rock JA and Jones HW Jr: The clinical management of the double uterus, Fertil Steril 28:798, 1977.
26. Rock JA: Resectoscopic techniques for the lysis of a Class V complete uterine septum, Fertil Steril 48:495, 1987.
27. Siegler AM: Hysterosalpingography, New York, 1967, Hoeber Medical Division, Harper & Row.
28. Valle RF and Sciarra JJ: Hysteroscopic treatment of the septate uterus, Obstet Gynecol 67:253, 1986.

# 6 *Intrauterine Adhesions*

Hysteroscopy is the most reliable diagnostic method for detecting intrauterine adhesions. Lysis of these adhesions using hysteroscopic control is the method preferred to restore normal intrauterine architecture.

## ETIOLOGY

More than 90% of patients who develop intrauterine adhesions (IUAs) have had a curettage in conjunction with pregnancy. About one third of IUAs develop following curettage for evacuation of an incomplete spontaneous abortion and another third after elective termination of pregnancy.[12] The endometrium, however, seems most vulnerable to injury during the early postpartum phase (the first 3 weeks). A curettage done to control bleeding during this time usually results in the formation of IUAs. There appears to be no difference in occurrence between nursing and nonnursing mothers. Adoni et al.[1] found that adhesions occurred more often after curettage for missed abortion than curettage necessitated for an incomplete abortion. Adhesions were observed in 42 women, 13 (30.9%) who had a missed abortion compared with 78 patients, only 5 (6.4%) of whom had an early abortion. A delivery by cesarean section rarely causes intrauterine adhesions. If IUAs do develop following cesarean section, they are the result of inadvertent sutures to apposing uterine walls. Tuberculous endometritis results in severe distortion of the uterine shadow during hysterography and causes associated amenorrhea and intrauterine adhesions. Occasionally this condition has been seen following a metroplasty, a submucous myomectomy, and a diagnostic curettage. The routine use of curettage for an infertile patient during a diagnostic laparoscopy is unwarranted because it can lead to the formation of IUAs and provides minimal information for the physician.

## SYMPTOMS AND SIGNS

Amenorrhea, hypomenorrhea, and repeated abortions are the main symptoms of intrauterine adhesions. Over 75% of women with moderate to severe adhesions will have either amenorrhea or hypomenorrhea. Cyclic abdominal pain at the time of the expected menses and the failure to menstruate may indicate atretic traumatic amenorrhea.[3] The endometrial cavity above the constricted or stenotic isthmus could have normally functioning endometrium, but the lower segment has no opening to allow the exit of menstrual blood. A hematometra can result followed by the uncommon complication of hematosalpinx. Intrauterine adhesions are discovered in patients who have normal menses because the HSG done during an infertility investigation reveals suspicious intrauterine defects that are subsequently confirmed by hysteroscopy. Therefore the possibility of IUAs cannot be excluded even for women who have cyclic, painless menses with a normal flow. Asherman[4] termed this condition *traumatic intrauterine adhesions.*

## DIAGNOSIS

The history of a curettage of a recently pregnant uterus followed by amenorrhea or hypomenorrhea is very significant. The combination of these two facts should lead the physician to suspect the diagnosis of IUA. If the patient desires to become pregnant, a simple method used to ascertain ovarian function is recording basal temperature on a chart. A biphasic pattern in the absence of menses indicates IUA. Withdrawal bleeding usually does not occur following cyclic administration of estrogen and progesterone to stimulate the growth of the scarred endometrial surface. Withdrawal bleeding indicates some residual, viable endometrium and therefore a better prognosis.

A uterine sound can ascertain the depth of the cavity or the presence of a constriction in the lower uterine segment. In the latter instance, the release of old dark blood almost confirms the diagnosis.

### Hysterosalpingography

About 5% of all patients on whom HSGs are performed for treatment of repeat abortions will show IUA. HSGs will reveal the condition in 39% of the patients with a history compatible with IUA, but are found unexpectedly in only 1%. Suspected intrauterine adhesions are diagnosed in a hysterogram that reveals filling defects, in an often smaller than normal uterine cavity, that has irregular, ragged contours. The lacunar-like defects have sharp borders and tend to persist as additional increments of contrast medium are added. The slow instillation of the medium under image intensified fluoroscopy, with spot films taken at propitious moments of uterine filling, is essential for an adequate study. This technique also detects evidence of early vascular intravasation seen in some women. It is uncommon for the patient to have a normal hysterogram and for significant, focal agglutination of the uterine cavity to be detected by hysteroscopy. Clinically insignificant endometrial adhesions can exist, however, with a normal uterine shadow. Hysterography remains the definitive diagnostic procedure used to screen patients for IUA. Although a normal uterine shadow can exclude the diagnosis, intrauterine defects interpreted as adhesions are sometimes not confirmed at hysteroscopy either, and other possible intrauterine abnormalities can be found.

The type and degree of adhesions cannot be established with certainty by hysterography. In a series of hysterograms, 80 were interpreted as revealing severe involvement. Hysteroscopy revealed mild involvement for 4 cases, and 23 others revealed moderate adhesions. The findings of the remaining 53 were the same as the hysterographic findings. Of the 54 hysterograms showing minimal to moderate uterine involvement, all but 5 revealed the same information as the x-ray interpretation.[17] Cervical stenosis caused by agglutination at the internal os or lower uterine segment can result in amenorrhea. The hysterogram shows the lower uterine segment only as a finger-like projection. The uterine cavity above can be quite normal, and removal of the constriction or agglutination will result in the release of old dark blood.

## Ultrasonography

Early secretory and late proliferative endometrium can be evaluated sonographically. A sonolucent symmetrical line appears when the endometrium proliferates, and a small amount of fluid separates the uterine walls. Such a finding is typical when the endometrium is stimulated by an excessive amount of estrogen. The sonographic appearance of IUA clearly differs from such a picture. IUAs are echogenic rather than sonolucent, and their location is usually asymmetrical within the uterine cavity.[5,26]

Confino et al.[6] described sonographic imaging of IUAs that gave an echogenic appearance and were asymmetrically placed within the uterine cavities of three patients. The sonographic disappearance of the structure after lysis of the adhesions supports the contention that abnormal intrauterine sonographic echogenicity indicates the presence of IUA.

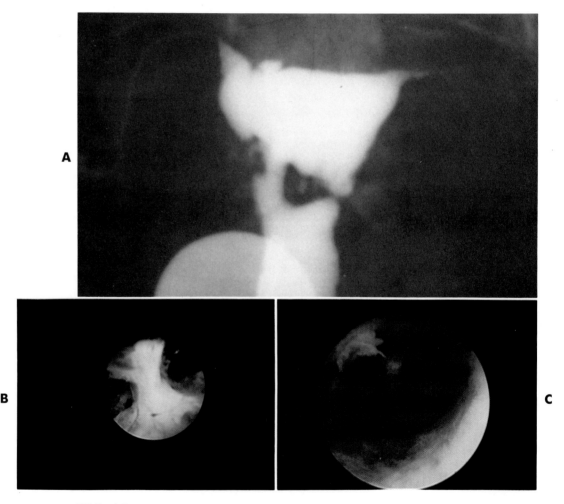

*FIG. 6-1* **A,** HSG shows filling defect with irregular borders in lower part of uterine cavity. **B,** Single thick adhesion is seen. **C,** Adhesion has been removed.

## Hysteroscopy

Hysteroscopy can reveal central adhesions that appear as vertical or oblique columns and marginal crescent-shaped adhesions that obscure the corresponding cornu. It can ascertain the size of the adhesions and evaluate the surrounding endometrium. Hysteroscopy has several advantages over an HSG; the synechiae can be located more precisely, lysis can be performed under direct vision, and the value of therapy can be ascertained in a follow-up hysteroscopic diagnostic examination (Figs. 6-1 and 6-2).[8,21]

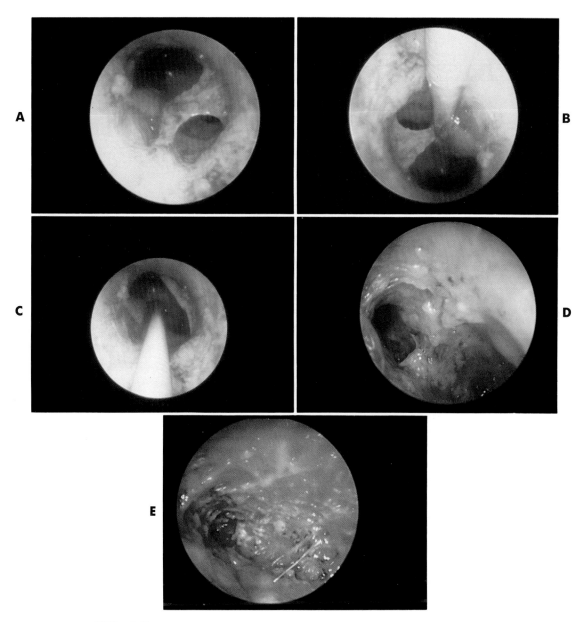

*FIG. 6-2*  **A,** Thick central adhesive band is noted. **B,** Band is divided. **C,** Edges of adhesion are seen with normal uterine cavity in background. **D,** Central adhesion is present. **E,** Thin fundal adhesions are seen.

## CLASSIFICATIONS

Classifications currently used are based on the hysterographic[24] and hysteroscopic[16] appearance of the intrauterine adhesions and their histology.[10]

### Hysterographic Classifications

IUAs have a characteristic appearance on the HSG but vary greatly in location and extent. Filling defects usually are seen within the uterine cavity and cause partial obliteration of the cavity at certain points where the anterior and posterior walls fuse. Most adhesions are in the fundus and allow the introduction of contrast fluid for diagnosis. Occasionally IUAs may obliterate the entire uterine cavity or obstruct the lower uterine segment and permit opacification of only a short segment of a blunt-ending cervical canal. Hysterographic classifications were devised to assess the impact of these diverse pictures and compare them to subsequent hysteroscopic findings and reproductive outcomes postoperatively.

*Mild*

Multiple, linear intrauterine defects are usually centrally located, and they cause minimal distortion of the uterine outline. Less than one third of the cavity is involved (Fig. 6-3).

*Moderate*

The borders of the uterine shadow are irregular and have multiple lacunar defects. About two thirds of the cavity is involved (Fig. 6-4).

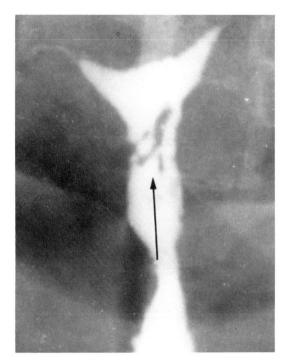

*FIG. 6-3* Multiple small central filling defects are seen and represent mild IUA.

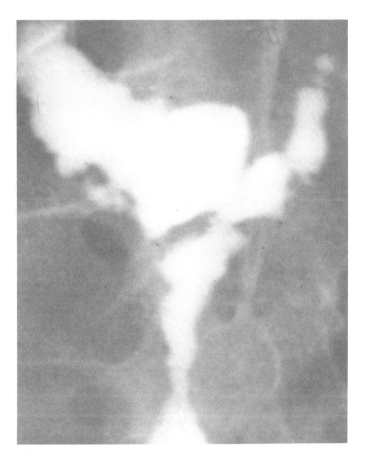

*FIG. 6-4* Irregular uterine borders involving more than one half of uterine cavity were caused by moderate IUA.

*Severe*

The uterine shadow is completely distorted, especially in the fundus, with evidence of myometrial and vascular intravasation. Tubal occlusion is often present (Fig. 6-5). In other instances only the lower segment can be filled with contrast fluid because the remainder of the cavity is obliterated by uterine synechiae. Hematometra does not occur despite occlusion of the endocervical canal. Presumably, the remaining endometrium either becomes refractory to hormonal stimuli or has been replaced by fibrous tissue.

For some patients suffering from severe menometrorrhagia, HSGs done 3 to 6 months after endometrial ablation using the Nd:YAG laser will indicate severe IUAs. Ostensibly, the coagulation necrosis that results from photocoagulation and possibly the associated carbonization, predispose these women to intrauterine adhesions. Postoperative hysteroscopic examinations show extensive IUAs. Following endometrial ablation, HSGs that involve the use of electrosurgical resection or roller ball coagulation reveal a small but normal uterine contour. During hysteroscopy the cavity appears smooth.

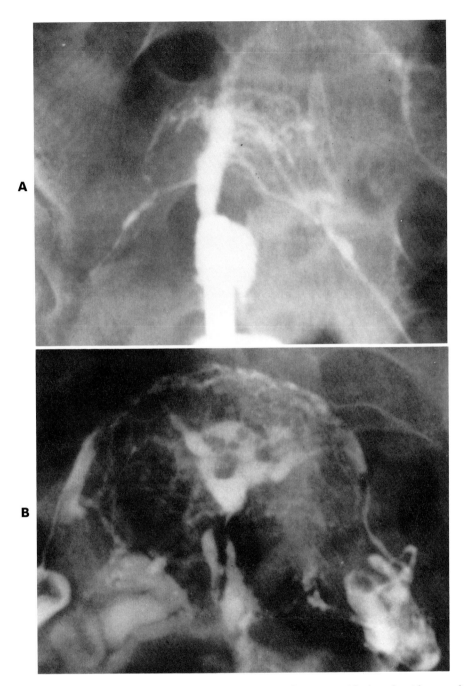

*FIG. 6-5* **A,** Small part of uterine cavity has been opacified and evidence of vascular intravasation is noted. **B,** Similar HSG is seen with some tubal filling. Severe intrauterine adhesions are illustrated.

### Hysteroscopic Classifications

One hysteroscopic classification of adhesions is based on the degree of occlusion of the uterine cavity especially in the ostial and fundal areas.[16,17]

This classification consists of three categories and depends on whether adhesions make up one fourth, one half, or three fourths of the uterine cavity. The clinician can approximate the extent of the cavitary lesion and is permitted a basis for comparing the hysteroscopy with the HSG. To analyze the results of treatment, a postoperative hysteroscopic procedure done in the office is preferable to an HSG because it is more accurate and quite easily performed. The HSG is primarily a screening procedure, which detects instances of intrauterine filling defects that can be more precisely evaluated endoscopically.

*Minimal*

Less than one fourth of the uterine cavity contains filmy adhesions, but ostial areas and upper fundus are minimally involved or clear (Fig. 6-6).

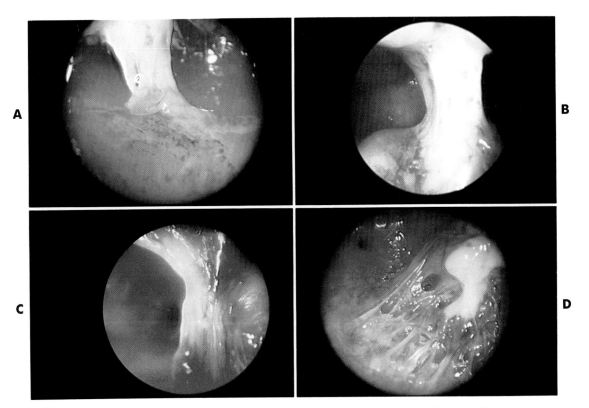

*FIG. 6-6* **A,** Central endometrial adhesion is seen. **B,** Thick fibrous adhesion simulates septum. Fundus is seen in background. **C,** Single adhesion is illustrated. **D,** Multiple, thin endometrial adhesions are present.

*Moderate*

Almost three fourths of the uterine cavity shows adhesion involvement, but the walls are not agglutinated. The ostial areas and upper fundus are partially occluded (Fig. 6-7).

*Severe*

More than three fourths of the uterine cavity contains thick bands. There is agglutination of uterine walls, and ostial areas, and the upper cavity are involved (Fig. 6-8).

It is sometimes difficult to evaluate the extent of endometrial cavity obliteration because the view of the region above the adhesions is restricted.

The HSG tends to exaggerate the extent of the disease and often indicates less severe adhesive disease than hysteroscopy does. As expected, there is a correlation between the extent of adhesions and the menstrual pattern. Most patients who complain of amenorrhea or hypomenorrhea have severe adhesions, although on rare occasions, normal menses occur in patients who have extensive intrauterine synechiae.

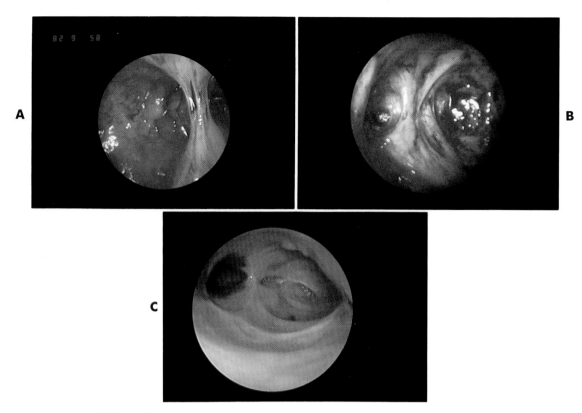

FIG. 6-7 A, Moderate IUAs obscure one cornual area. B, Severe adhesions are present, and only one uterotubal orifice is seen. C, Only part of one uterine horn is seen, other is obscured by adhesions.

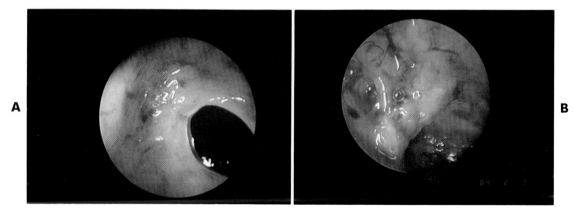

FIG. 6-8 A, Extensive, wide IUA has obliterated most of upper uterine cavity. B, Previous failed attempt at hysteroscopic lysis resulted in distorted uterine cavity without any distinct landmarks.

## Histologic Classifications

Hamou et al.[10] described three types of IUA at × 20 magnification.

1. Endometrial adhesions appeared white with some glandular and vascular patterns similar to those of the surrounding endometrium. They were easily dissected.
2. Synechiae composed of either fibrous or connective tissue appeared transparent, thin, bridgelike, were poorly vascularized, formed stumps after lysis, and usually their position was central or isthmic.
3. Myometrial adhesions limited uterine distention, general anesthesia was required for lysis. The fibrous adhesions were more common in moderate adhesions. The location of adhesions of the endometrial type was usually central, and they had been there less than 1 year. Often myometrial adhesions were more extensive and had been there longer. Based on these findings Hamou et al.,[10] suggested the following classifications.

### Mild

Endometrial adhesions are filmy, avascular, and easily disrupted.

### Moderate

Fibromuscular adhesions are characteristically thick but may be covered by endometrium and can bleed when divided.

### Severe

Connective or fibrous tissue adhesions lack any endometrial lining and do not bleed when divided.

All three types can partially or completely obliterate the uterine cavity.

The American Fertility Society[2] has proposed a classification of intrauterine adhesions based on the hysteroscopic findings of the extent of the cavity involved, the type of adhesions, and the menstrual pattern. Its adoption could mean standardized reports; therefore more meaningful comparison of results could be made. Points are given for each stage of the disease: mild, moderate, or severe, and their summation provides a score (Fig. 6-9).

# THE AMERICAN FERTILITY SOCIETY CLASSIFICATION OF INTRAUTERINE ADHESIONS

Patient's Name _____ Date _____ Chart # _____

Age _____ G _____ P _____ Sp Ab _____ VTP _____ Ectopic _____ Infertile Yes _____ No _____

Other Significant History (i.e. surgery, infection, etc.) _____

_____

HSG _____ Sonography _____ Photography _____ Laparoscopy _____ Laparotomy _____

| Extent of<br>Cavity Involved | <1/3 | 1/3 - 2/3 | >2/3 |
|---|---|---|---|
| | 1 | 2 | 4 |
| Type of<br>Adhesions | Filmy | Filmy & Dense | Dense |
| | 1 | 2 | 4 |
| Menstrual<br>Pattern | Normal | Hypomenorrhea | Amenorrhea |
| | 0 | 2 | 4 |

**Prognostic Classification**

| | | | HSG*<br>Score | Hysteroscopy<br>Score |
|---|---|---|---|---|
| Stage I | (Mild) | 1-4 | _____ | _____ |
| Stage II | (Moderate) | 5-8 | _____ | _____ |
| Stage III | (Severe) | 9-12 | _____ | _____ |

*All adhesions should be considered dense

**Treatment (Surgical Procedures):** _____

_____

_____

_____

_____

**Prognosis for Conception & Subsequent Viable Infant***

_____ Excellent ( > 75% )

_____ Good ( 50-75% )

_____ Fair ( 25%-50% )

_____ Poor ( < 25% )

*Physician's judgment based upon tubal patency.

**Recommended Followup Treatment:** _____

_____

_____

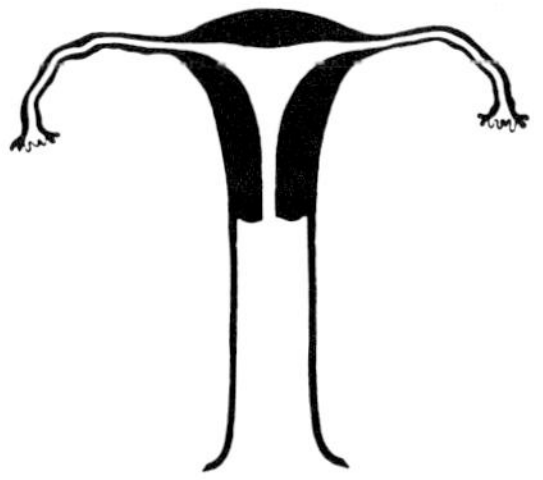

Property of
The American Fertility Society

**Additional Findings:** _____

_____

_____

_____

_____

**DRAWING**

**HSG Findings**

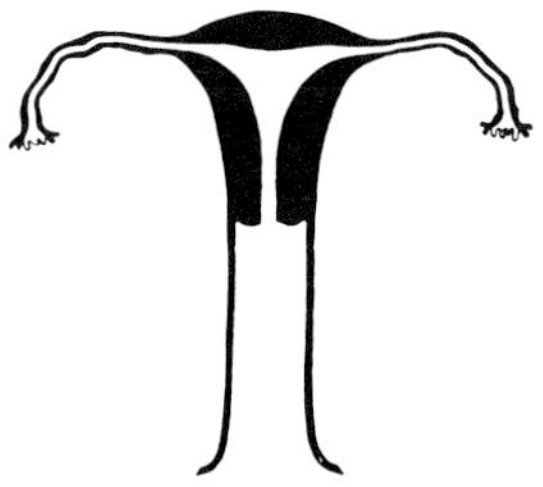

**Hysteroscopy Findings**

For additional supply write to:
The American Fertility Society
2140 11th Avenue, South
Suite 200
Birmingham, Alabama 35205

*FIG. 6-9* Classification of intrauterine adhesions proposed by American Fertility Society. From The American Fertility Society: The American Fertility Society classifications of adnexal adhesions, distal tubal occlusion, tubal occlusion secondary to tubal ligation, tubal pregnancies, Müllerian anomalies and intrauterine adhesions. Fertil Steril 49:944, 1988. Reproduced with permission of the publisher, The American Fertility Society.

## THERAPY

Hysteroscopy has been used increasingly to diagnose and manage intrauterine abnormalities so it is quite natural to use it to treat intrauterine adhesions. Since the presence of moderate to severe intrauterine adhesions can mean a serious prognosis, they should be lysed with care by an experienced hysteroscopist, and the obstetric care given must be planned with consideration for potential complications.

The selection of a patient for dissection of intrauterine adhesions should be based on hysteroscopic confirmation of the disease. Although a curettage related to pregnancy is evident for over 90% of these women, other causes of induced trauma to the endometrial lining can result in IUA. The patient who has experienced multiple pregnancy losses also requires additional study to rule out contributing factors. Important screening procedures include cervical cultures for chlamydia, thyroid function studies, and karyotyping of the couple.

The therapeutic principles include the restoration of the normal uterine architecture, prevention of the recurrence of adhesions, and the promotion of endometrial regeneration. Preoperatively, patients are informed that sometimes more than one procedure may be required. The postoperative regimen is described carefully.

Simultaneous laparoscopy is advised when:

1. The HSG indicates venous intravasation or tubal occlusion
2. A fine probe cannot be introduced into the uterine cavity
3. The diagnostic hysteroscopy reveals extensive lateral synechiae and the ostial areas are occluded
4. No landmarks (i.e., cornua, tubal ostia) are visible after considerable dissection. Laparoscopic control guided by the surgeon helps avoid uterine perforation. The fiberoptic light is turned down during the laparoscopy procedure to allow observation of the proximity of the hysteroscopic dissection to the uterine serosal surface.

## Hysteroscopy

Lysis of synechiae under hysteroscopic control is safer and more complete than "blind" curettage or hysterotomy. Using accessory instruments it is possible to cut the scar tissue and limit the trauma to the normal endometrium. In patients who continue to menstruate in spite of IUA, hysteroscopy is performed during the follicular phase using a 7 mm operative sheath with either a 0° or 30° hysteroscope. In women who have minimal or moderate disease, a local paracervical block and intravenous meperidine or diazepam (Valium) minimize the discomfort from the dissection. A general anesthesia is required for removal of severe adhesions suggested by the hysterogram or previous office hysteroscopy.

All of the media used for uterine distention have been successful during lysis of IUA. Observation begins at the internal os, and adhesions in that area are divided before the endoscope is advanced. The uterine cavity is sculptured systematically until symmetry is achieved. When adhesions are focal, they are divided but removal is not attempted. As the adhesions are cut, the stumps retract, the uterine cavity distends, and both cornu and uterotubal ostia should come into view. Marginal adhesions are often composed of fibromuscular and connective tissues, and careful dissection is required to avoid uterine perforation. Simultaneous laparoscopy, without the fiberoptic light, reveals the transillumination of the uterine cavity as the dissection is monitored. Chromopertubation can be attempted in selected instances while the laparoscope is in place.

Various hysteroscopic techniques have been described. In 1974 Edström[7] used the sharp distal end of the endoscope to rupture the adhesions in 9 patients and excised some tissue with biopsy forceps. Levine and Neuwirth[15] inserted either miniature scissors or an electrosurgical probe to coagulate and cut adhesions through the accessory channel of the sheath. Sugimoto[25] used the outer sleeve of the hysteroscope to break central adhesions. For marginal adhesions, a Kelly forceps was used with a follow-up hysteroscopy to evaluate the completeness of the procedure. Hamou et al.[10] called their technique *target abrasion* as adhesions were disrupted by the beveled end of the hysteroscope and sheath. The semirigid scissors, however, can be manipulated more precisely, and, occasionally, rigid fixed optic scissors are used for focal adhesions because an unimpeded panoramic view is essential. The modified urologic resectoscope also has been used successfully to shave adhesions electrosurgically.[19] Lasers (Nd:YAG, argon, KTP/532)[27] delivered through quartz fibers have been used to divide adhesions, but their actions may damage normal remaining endometrium because of lateral and frontal scatter. The sapphire tip of the Nd:YAG laser can cut with less scattering. The value of lasers in the surgical management of IUAs requires further clinical evaluation.

Adhesiolysis rather than total excision is a satisfactory surgical procedure. Each adhesive band is identified and divided with miniature scissors. The operation seldom causes significant bleeding except when the myometrium is reached (Figs. 6-10 and 6-11). Hysteroscopic adhesiolysis combined with hysterography has been advocated by Lancet and Mass[14] and adapted to fluoroscopy by Wamsteker.[28] This approach may be warranted for patients who have severe obliteration of the endometrial cavity particularly in the fundal area, with an impaired view of the uterine cavity despite tubal patency.

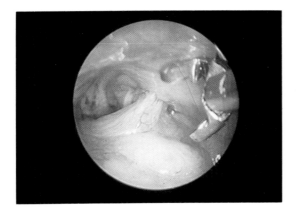

*FIG. 6-10* Extensive fundal adhesions are divided under hysteroscopic control.

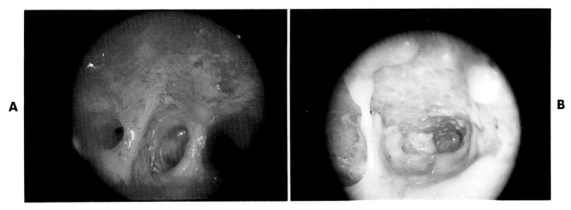

*FIG. 6-11* **A,** Severe intrauterine adhesions have covered upper portion of uterine cavity. **B,** Under hysteroscopic control, adhesions have been carefully cut, minimal bleeding is noted.

## Ancillary Therapy

An intrauterine splint, in the form of an IUD, has been advocated by most gynecologists in their postoperative management regimen to prevent recurrence of the adhesions. The IUD is inserted and retained for approximately 2 months. When the patient refuses an IUD, or the dissection is insufficient to enable placement, or if a uterine perforation is suspected, a No. 8 Fr foley catheter is inserted and the balloon filled with 3 ml of NS. The section of the catheter protruding through the external os is tied and the distal portion is removed. In the series of patients described by Hamou et al.,[10] 28 women who had small adhesions of less than 1-year's duration did not receive an IUD. Lippes IUDs (Ortho Pharmaceutical Corporation, Raritan, NJ) were inserted in 41 patients. The selection of these patients was based on several factors. Eleven women had severe adhesions, 12 had adhesions for at least 1 year, 9 had fibrous adhesions, 6 others had central adhesions, and 3 women showed reappearance of adhesions after the initial follow-up hysteroscopy. Although the Lippes loop has been used by many gynecologists, withdrawal of IUDs from the market in the United States has prompted the use of an alternative such as the No. 8 Fr foley balloon catheter.

Despite the absence of randomized studies on the prospective value of prophylactic antibiotics, they are suggested because of the need for intrauterine surgery, the great interest of these patients in fertility, and postoperative insertion of an IUD. Antibiotics are advised 1 hour before treatment and for 2 or 3 postoperative doses. Whenever the intrauterine catheter is used, antibiotic treatment is advised until the device is removed.

Conjugated estrogens, 5 mg daily, are prescribed for 60 consecutive days to build up the endometrium, and, on the final 10 days, medroxyprogesterone acetate, 10 mg daily, is added to differentiate the endometrium and bring about sloughing. Spotting can sometimes occur during the estrogen therapy, but the dose is increased only if the bleeding is heavy. The IUD and hormones are prescribed for patients with moderate and severe disease who have associated menstrual dysfunction such as hypomenorrhea and amenorrhea. They are not advocated in patients who have a single adhesion or multiple, thin central adhesions and whose endometrial lining appears well preserved. Shortly before the therapy is stopped, the IUD is removed.

## COMPLICATIONS

The main intraoperative complication is the occurrence of a uterine perforation. If the hysteroscopic procedure is performed under laparoscopic control, this accident should not cause any sequelae. The operation can be completed, providing uterine distention can be maintained. The insertion of the IUD should be done under laparoscopic control to prevent its inadvertent passage intraabdominally. Patients should be informed of complications. If pregnancy occurs postoperatively, the obstetrician can be made aware of this circumstance, and the pregnancy managed accordingly.

Intraoperative hemorrhage is rare but excessive bleeding can be controlled by the use of a No. 8 Fr foley balloon catheter for a few days. In these cases the intrauterine adhesions can be severe, and an intraoperative complication can occur. The endometrium tends to renew itself on a monthly basis, but in some instances the basal layer is replaced with scar tissue. The basalis from the adjacent or unscarred endometrium does not migrate laterally to cover the scarred area. Intravascular intravasation, during the preoperative HSG, may indicate a scarred or absent basal layer. This condition is seen even after the release of the adhesions and indicates a residual endometrial abnormality.

Reports of obstetric complications in a subsequent pregnancy include placenta accreta, intrauterine sacculation, and even uterine dehiscence.[11] Of 187 patients treated hysteroscopically by Valle and Sciarra,[27] only one pregnant woman subsequently developed a partial placenta accreta. Friedman et al.[9] described three obstetric sequelae following adhesiolysis in 33 patients. One of these was a placenta increta; another woman developed a large sacculation in the posterior lower uterine segment. In this latter case a uterine perforation followed the placement of an IUD to maintain the shape of the uterine cavity. A third complication was a uterine dehiscence discovered at a cesarean birth, but the patient had a cesarean before developing Asherman's syndrome.

Restoration of menstruation or even fertility after treatment for IUA is not followed necessarily by a normal obstetric outcome. Placenta accreta reported in almost 8% of the patients is the most serious complication, and it is caused by the lack of the decidua basalis at the site of the intrauterine adhesions. A repeat abortion rate of 25% and premature labor in 9% result from either recurrence of the IUA, endometrial insufficiency, or scarring.[27]

## RESULTS

After completing the procedure and postoperative therapy, the patient should have a diagnostic hysteroscopic examination in the office to evaluate the results. In women whose preoperative HSG showed tubal obstruction, a repeat HSG is advisable to ascertain whether the dissection of the cornual and ostial adhesions have resulted in tubal patency.

Extensive reviews of the diagnosis of IUAs, their management, and the results of therapy have been published.[13,22] Valle and Sciarra[27] wrote that removal of mild, filmy adhesions in 43 patients was followed by 35 (81%) term pregnancies; 97 moderate cases of fibromuscular adhesions showed 64 (66%) term pregnancies; and 47 cases with severe connective tissue adhesions resulted in 15 (32%) term pregnancies. Overall restoration of menses occurred in 90%, and the term pregnancy rate was 61%. Of 175 patients reported by March,[17] 69 wanted to become pregnant and had no other infertility factors. Fifty-two (75%) had 62 pregnancies, 54 (87%) going to term. Of 104 patients who complained of amenorrhea, 100 developed normal menses postoperatively, 4 others had hypomenorrhea, and only 1 of these 4 had persistent amenorrhea. These results give the impression that the treatment has improved with the advent of hysteroscopy since pregnancy rate results in earlier series were not as good.[18,20,23] An alternate explanation might be that the denominator has changed because milder cases included in recent series are detected by hysteroscopy. Other factors influencing the results following hysteroscopic lysis of IUA are the exclusion of patients who did not wish to become pregnant or those who had other infertility problems. As one reviews the many reports on this subject, it becomes quite clear that results are difficult to compare because of a lack of uniform classifications for intrauterine adhesions.

What is the measure of a successful outcome? Restoration of menses in a patient who previously has had amenorrhea or hypomenorrhea is one objective of therapy. Reports of the percentage of patients who achieve a pregnancy postoperatively can be misleading in women whose problem may have been repeated abortions. An uncomplicated term pregnancy should be considered the ultimate measure of success (Table 6-1).

*Table 6-1* Hysteroscopic Lysis of Intrauterine Adhesions

| Author | Cases (No.) | Medium Used | Technique | Menses | | Reproductive Outcome | | | |
|---|---|---|---|---|---|---|---|---|---|
| | | | | | | Pregnancy | | Term | |
| | | | | No. | % | No. | % | No. | % |
| Levine/Neuwirth[15] | 10 | Hyskon | Flexible scissors | 5 | 50 | 2 | 20 | 1 | 11 |
| Edström[7] | 9 | Hyskon | Target abrasion/biopsy forceps | 2 | 22 | 1 | 11 | 1 | 11 |
| Siegler/Kontopoulos[24] | 25 | $CO_2$ | Target abrasion/curettage/scissors | 13 | 52 | 11 | 44 | 12 | 44.4 |
| March/Israel[16] | 38 | Hyskon | Flexible scissors | 38 | 100 | 38 | 100 | 34 | 79.1 |
| Neuwirth et al.[18] | 27 | Hyskon | Scissors along side of hysteroscope | 20 | 74 | 14 | 51.8 | 13 | 48.1 |
| Sanfilippo et al.[21] | 26 | $CO_2$ | Curettage | 26 | 100 | 6 | 100 | 3 | 50 |
| Hamou et al.[10] | 69 | $CO_2$ | Target abrasion | 59 | 85.5 | 20 | 51.3 | 15 | 38.4 |
| Sugimoto et al.[25] | 258 | Hyskon/NS | Target abrasion/forceps | 180 | 69.9 | 143 | 76.4 | 114 | 79.7 |
| Wamsteker[28] | 36 | Hyskon | Scissors/biopsy forceps | 34 | 94.4 | 17 | 62.9 | 12 | 44.4 |
| Friedman et al.[9] | 30 | Hyskon | Resectoscope/scissors | 27 | 90 | 24 | 80 | 23 | 76.6 |
| Zuanchong/Yulian[29] | 70 | $D_5W$ | Biopsy forceps/scissors | 64 | 84.3 | 30 | 85.7 | 17 | 48.5 |
| Valle/Sciarra[27] | 187 | Hyskon/$D_5W$ | Semirigid scissors | 167 | 89.3 | 143 | 76.4 | 114 | 79.7 |
| Lancet/Kessler[13] | 98 | ? | Scissors | 98 | 100 | 86 | 87.8 | 77 | 89.5 |
| TOTALS | 883*† | | | 773 | 83.0 | 535 | 60.5 | 435 | 81.3‡ |

*All authors used estrogens, progestogens, and IUDs postoperatively.
†Prophylactic antibiotics were used in 50% of the patients.
‡Based on the number of pregnant patients; based on the number of patients treated the percentage of term pregnancies is 49% (435/883).

## References

1. Adoni AS, Palti Z, Milwidsky A, et al.: The incidence of intrauterine adhesions following spontaneous abortion, Int J Fertil 27:117, 1982.

2. American Fertility Society: The American Fertility Society classification of adnexal adhesions, distal tubal occlusion, tubal occlusion secondary to tubal ligation, tubal pregnancies, müllerian anomalies and intrauterine adhesions, Fertil Steril 49:944, 1988.

3. Asherman JG: Amenorrhea traumatica (atretica), J Obstet Gynaecol Br Emp 55:23, 1948.

4. Asherman JG: Traumatic intrauterine adhesions, J Obstet Gynaecol Br Emp 57:892, 1950.

5. Bouton M and Denhez M: Les modifications de la muqueuse endometriale à l'echographie: influences hormonales et endometriales, Contraception, Fertil Sexual 11:235, 1983.

6. Confino E, Friberg J, Giglia RV, and Gleicher N: Sonographic imaging of intrauterine adhesions, Obstet Gynecol 66:596, 1985.

7. Edström KGB: Intrauterine surgical procedures during hysteroscopy, Endoscopy 6:175, 1974.

8. Fayez JA, Mutie G, and Schneider PJ: The diagnostic value of hysterosalpingography and hysteroscopy in infertility investigation, Am J Obstet Gynecol 156:558, 1987.

9. Friedman A, Defazio J, and DeCherney AH: Severe obstetric complications following hysteroscopic lysis of adhesions, Obstet Gynecol 67:864, 1986.

10. Hamou J, Salat-Baroux J, and Siegler AM: Diagnosis and treatment of intrauterine adhesions by microhysteroscopy, Fertil Steril 39:321, 1983.

11. Jewelewicz R, Khalaf S, Neuwirth RS, and Vande Wiele RL: Obstetric complications after treatment of intrauterine synechiae (Asherman's syndrome), Obstet Gynecol 47:701, 1976.

12. Kremer J, Hamou J, and Salat-Baroux J: Aspects hystéroscopiques dans les suites d'interruptions volontaires de grossesse, Paris, 1980, Thése Facul de Med de Paris.

13. Lancet M and Kessler I: A review of Asherman's syndrome, and results of modern treatment, Int J Fertil 33:14, 1988.

14. Lancet M and Mass N: Concomitant hysterography and hysteroscopy in Asherman's syndrome, Int J Fertil 26:267, 1981.

15. Levine RU and Neuwirth RS: Simultaneous laparoscopy and hysteroscopy for intrauterine adhesions, Obstet Gynecol 42:441, 1973.

16. March CM and Israel R: Gestational outcome following hysteroscopic lysis of adhesions, Fertil Steril 36: 455, 1981.

17. March CM: Hysteroscopy and the uterine factor in infertility. In Mishell DR Jr and Davajan V, eds: Infertility, contraception, and reproductive endocrinology, Oradell, NJ, 1986, Medical Economics Books.

18. Musset R and Netter A: Synechies utérines, Encyclopedie Gynecol Paris 10:140, 1972.

19. Neuwirth RS, Hussein AR, Schiffman BM, and Amin HK: Hysteroscopic resection of intrauterine scars using a new technique, Obstet Gynecol 60:111, 1982.

20. Oelsner G et al.: Outcome of pregnancy after treatment of intrauterine adhesions, Obstet Gynecol 44:341, 1974.

21. Sanfillipo JS, Fitzgerald MR, Badaway SZ, and Yussman MA: Asherman's syndrome: a comparison of methods, J Reprod Med 27:328, 1982.

22. Schenker JG and Margalioth EJ: Intrauterine adhesions: an updated appraisal, Fertil Steril 37:593, 1982.

23. Siegler AM and Kemmann EK: Hysteroscopy, Obstet Gynecol Surv 30: 567, 1975.

24. Siegler AM and Kontopoulos VG: Lysis of intrauterine adhesions under hysteroscopic control: A report of 25 operations, J Reprod Med 26: 372, 1981.

25. Sugimoto O, Ushiroyama T, and Fukuda Y: Diagnostic and therapeutic hysteroscopy for traumatic intrauterine adhesions. In Siegler AM and Lindemann HJ, eds: Hysteroscopy: principles and practice, Philadelphia, 1984, JB Lippincott.

26. Taylor KJW: Gynecology: atlas of ultrasonography, ed 2, New York, 1985, Churchill-Livingstone.

27. Valle RF and Sciarra JJ: Intrauterine adhesions: hysteroscopic diagnosis, classification, treatment, and reproductive outcome, Am J Obstet Gynecol 158:1459, 1988.

28. Wamsteker K: Hysteroscopy in Asherman's syndrome. In Siegler AM and Lindemann HJ, eds: Hysteroscopy: principles and practice, Philadelphia, 1984, JB Lippincott.

29. Zuanchong F and Yulian H: Hysteroscopic diagnosis and treatment of intrauterine adhesions: clinical analysis of 70 cases, Symposium on Hysteroscopy, Shanghai, 1986, Family Planning Association.

# 7 *Hysteroscopy and the IUD*

The position of a large proportion of occult intrauterine devices (IUDs) appears reversed within the uterine cavity (Fig. 7-1).[3] Expulsion can be caused by intrauterine lesions, a congenital anomaly, or a submucous myoma. Depending on the IUD used, expulsions occur from 2 to 20 per 100 insertions. Most expulsions occur within the first year and decrease in frequency every year thereafter. The tail of the IUD can be pulled into the endometrial cavity because of malpositioned insertion, rotation of the IUD, or uterine enlargement caused by pregnancy or myomas. Retraction of the tail of the IUD, without rotation, happens more often with the Copper 7 (Cu-7) (Fig. 7-2). Complete or partial IUD translocation is secondary to uterine perforation. Consensus is that most accidents occur at the time of insertion.

When threads are not visible or palpable, a search must be done to locate the IUD. It may have fractured, penetrated, or perforated the uterine wall, or it may have been expelled. Uncertainty and the chance for pregnancy mean stress for the patient and cause concern for her physician. IUDs can be medicated (copper or steroid bearing), nonmedicated, or opened, linear, or closed. Threads or tails attached to IUDs make it easy to check their presence and facilitate their removal.

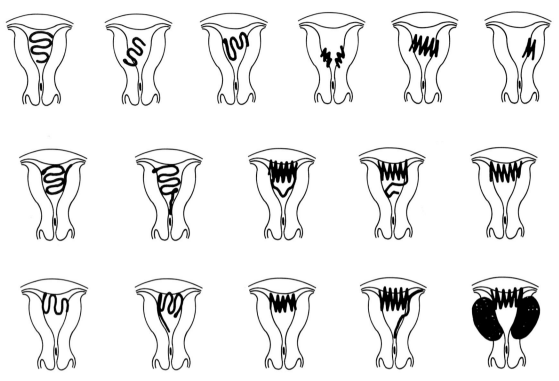

*FIG. 7-1* Schematic representation of IUDs in distorted positions within uterine cavity.

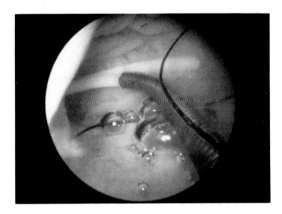

*FIG. 7-2* Cu-7 is normally placed within uterine cavity, but tail shown here has retracted.

Millen et al.[5] reviewed findings of 100 patients who had complained of "missing" strings. In half of them, the IUD had rotated, causing the string to be pulled into the cervix or uterine cavity. In 15 instances, the string had been cut too short. Twelve women became pregnant, four with the device in situ, and the device had been expelled in eight others. The device had been expelled in 13 nonpregnant women and were never located. The remaining 10 patients experienced uterine perforation. Nine devices were found in the peritoneal cavity and one IUD partially perforated the uterus. Uterine perforation occurs about once in every 2500 insertions, may be partial or complete, and should be suspected whenever the marker disappears from the external cervical os (Fig. 7-3, *A* and *B*). When complete perforation occurs, the ectopic IUD enters the peritoneal cavity and lies free in the posterior cul-de-sac or adheres to the uterus, adnexa, or peritoneum; it frequently becomes enmeshed in the omentum (Fig. 7-3, *C*).

Adel et al.[1] performed hysterography on 254 women, 2 years or more after an IUD had been inserted, to evaluate effects of prolonged use. In most symptomatic patients the device appeared to be distorted, the tip was partially embedded and molding of the uterine cavity was evident. Of women without complaints, 37% had similar radiographic findings. Tubal patency was seen in 87%. A recent report suggested that there are biochemical and cellular alterations in the composition of the tubal fluid causing premature lysis of the ovum.[2] Other possible tubal effects of the IUD cited were:

1. Accelerated transport of ova through the fallopian tubes
2. Failure of the oocyte to be picked up by the fimbria
3. Phagocytosis of spermatozoa by leukocytes in the tubal fluid

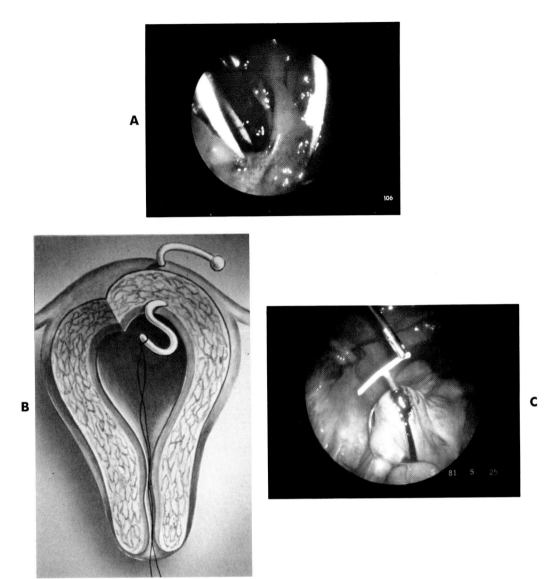

*FIG. 7-3* **A,** Spring device has penetrated myometrium. **B,** A section of the IUD has perforated the uterine cavity as shown. **C,** Device has passed through myometrium and is completely outside of uterine cavity.

## MANAGEMENT

Ultrasonography[6] and hysterography[3] can aid the search for the occult IUD, but use of the hysteroscope allows simultaneous detection and removal.[8-11] An x-ray film of the abdomen can indicate the presence of a radiopaque IUD, but offers no proof the device is intrauterine. If on the initial survey film the IUD is shown in the pelvis, before the next film is taken either a uterine sound or a second IUD is inserted and another exposure is made.

Hysterography can detect a possible or probable uterine perforation. It can reveal an IUD extending beyond the outline of a uterine cavity delineated with the contrast fluid (Fig. 7-4). The speculum should be removed before the films are taken to avoid obscuring the lower uterine segment, an area of possible perforation. The hysterogram can show an extrauterine position of the IUD and indicate various degrees of myometrial penetration. In one report, Rowe and McComb[7] described three patients who complained of primary infertility, but IUDs were seen on the hysterosalpingogram. These patients thought their IUDs had been removed.

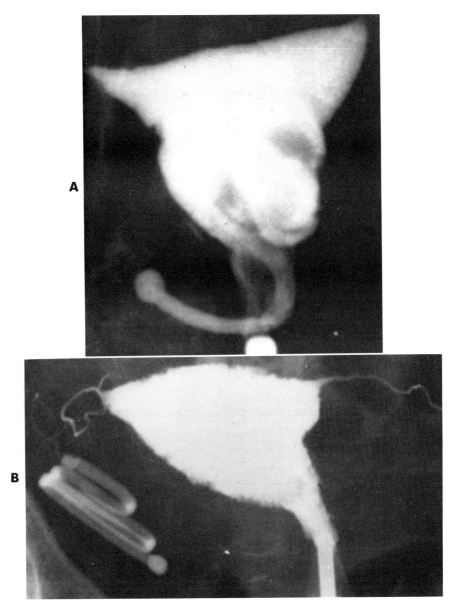

*FIG.* *7-4* **A,** IUD is in reversed position and upper part has penetrated lower uterine segment. **B,** HSG shows normal uterine cavity and extrauterine position of IUD.

The patient who complains that she cannot feel the cervical tail or the asymptomatic patient in whom the IUD tail cannot be discerned by speculum examination requires further study. A history should elicit the date of insertion, the type of IUD, pelvic pain or abnormal vaginal bleeding, date of failure to detect the IUD tail, the character of the last menses, and symptoms of pregnancy. During the pelvic examination the rectosigmoid area should be palpated to search for the translocated IUD in the cul-de-sac.

The endocervical canal should be explored initially with a cotton-tipped applicator to detect a shortened or slightly retracted thread. A tenaculum placed on the cervix followed by the introduction of a uterine sound can ascertain the length and direction of the cavity and "feel" the IUD. If the missing IUD is not found during these procedures, other diagnostic and therapeutic techniques are available.

Office hysteroscopy is one of those techniques. After a local anesthetic has been administered, a 5 mm diagnostic sheathed hysteroscope is inserted, and the uterine cavity is explored systematically. The IUD can be removed after its position has been located, using either a Novak curette, an alligator forceps, a retriever, or using a grasping forceps under hysteroscopic control (Fig. 7-5).

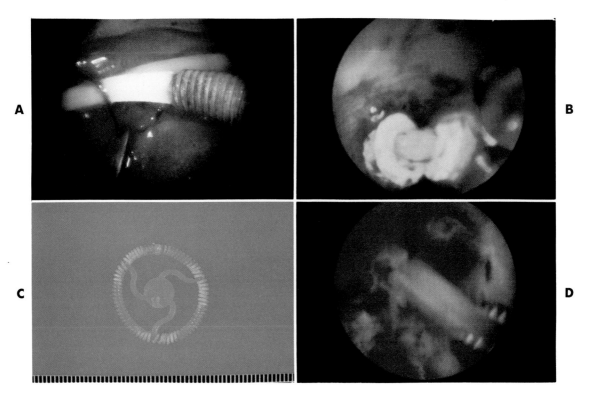

*FIG. 7-5*  **A,** Occult IUD was located in uterine cavity and grasped with forceps. **B,** Ota ring seen before removal. **C,** Removed Ota ring illustrated. **D,** Broken Dalkon shield found and removed under hysteroscopic control.

Fragments of plastic and metallic curettes, catheters, suture thread, splints, etc. that are dislodged or embedded in the uterine cavity have been successfully retrieved using hysteroscopic control when blind transcervical manipulation was not successful (Fig. 7-6).[14] If the IUD is correctly positioned, and its effectiveness has not been lost, it can be left in situ. The threads can be pulled into the cervical canal or extracted using hysteroscopic control (Fig. 7-7).

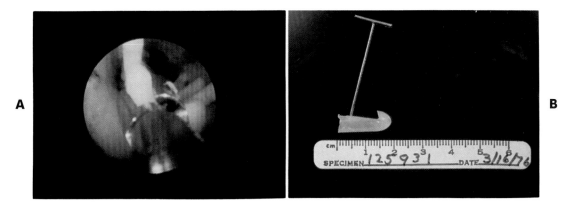

*FIG.* 7-6  **A,** Broken plastic tip located and removed by hysteroscopy. **B,** Specimen is seen.

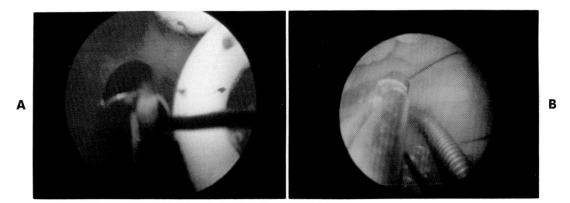

*FIG.* 7-7  **A,** Threads of IUDs can be grasped with forceps and **B,** subsequently pulled to external os.

If an IUD cannot be withdrawn easily through the vagina, persistent manipulation without implementing a hysterogram or hysteroscopy to locate its position can cause inadvertent trauma (Fig. 7-8). Once the extrauterine position of the IUD has been ascertained the patient must be informed. The decision to remove the IUD or to allow it to remain in situ must be made. Removal of an ectopic IUD is justified if the IUD is the possible source of the complications for the patient. IUDs can perforate neighboring viscera, particularly the rectosigmoid, small bowel, cecum, appendix, and rarely, the urinary bladder. Herniation, leading to incarceration and strangulation,[13] of a loop of small bowel can occur because of the interstice of a closed IUD. Such sequelae are rare.

Lippes,[4] citing an incidence of perforation of 0.1%, estimated there were about 30,000 ectopically located IUDs. Since complications from intraperitoneal linear devices are rare, it seems unjustified to subject 30,000 women to the risks involved with anesthesia and surgery. As a result of postoperative complications secondary to aggressive management to retrieve an unmedicated, linear device, two deaths have been reported. There is a definite need to remove IUDs with closed configurations or copper IUDs. Either exploratory laparotomy, laparoscopy, or colpotomy are used to remove these extrauterine IUDs. Hysteroscopic removal is reserved for the intrauterine misplaced or occult IUD, or an IUD that has partially perforated the myometrium.

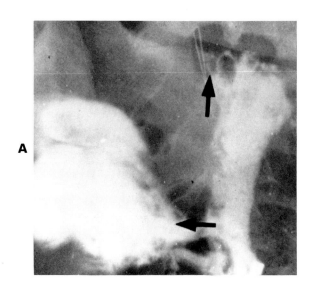

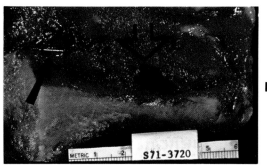

*FIG. 7-8* **A,** Following multiple attempts to remove fragment of IUD, HSG shows extravasation of contrast fluid into right broad ligament (*lower arrow*). *Upper arrow* points to fragment. **B,** Specimen shows uterine rupture in lower uterine segment (*open arrow*) and fragment of metallic IUD (*solid arrow*) in myometrium in fundus.

### Removal During Pregnancy

Instances that require hysteroscopic removal include unsuccessful attempts using conventional methods or when an IUD is associated with an intrauterine pregnancy. Excessive resistance to remove an IUD could be caused by a partial uterine perforation. Initial observation of the intrauterine position of the IUD is advised, and then a decision concerning the need for laparoscopic control is made (Fig. 7-9).

Tail retraction can be caused by an intrauterine pregnancy. To avoid a potential septic abortion, IUD extraction is advisable. If the pregnancy is allowed to continue, with the IUD in its proper position or an unknown position, the patient should be informed of the symptoms of a "sepsis-induced" abortion, which occurs frequently in the second trimester. A thorough examination of the placenta and membranes is made at delivery followed by manual exploration of the uterine cavity, if the IUD remains undetected. When the pregnancy is undesired an abortion is performed, and the IUD is often removed with the products of conception.

Alternatively, if the pregnancy is desired, or the patient objects to an induced abortion, an attempt is made to retrieve the IUD using hysteroscopy (Fig. 7-9). Hysteroscopy should be performed cautiously during pregnancy because an unplanned abortion can occur. Wagner[12] reported the results after removal of IUDs from 18 pregnant women under hysteroscopic control; in 14 patients the pregnancies remained intact. Valle[9] described 12 patients undergoing this procedure, 8 pregnancies went to term, 2 aborted spontaneously, and 2 patients developed significant bleeding during the procedure and immediate evacuation of the products of conception was required. New, smaller instruments have become available that permit hysteroscopic observation during pregnancy, and removal of the IUD is less traumatic.

If an IUD is located beneath the decidua near the nidation or is covered by the gestational sac, abortion is unavoidable. Patients must be made aware of this possibility. More data are needed concerning the risk of provoked abortion, the need for prophylactic antibiotics or hospitalization, and the possibility of heavy bleeding. Abortion does occur in 25% of the women who have an IUD removed, but if the IUD is allowed to remain in situ the abortion rate doubles, and the patient is at risk for a severe intrauterine infection.

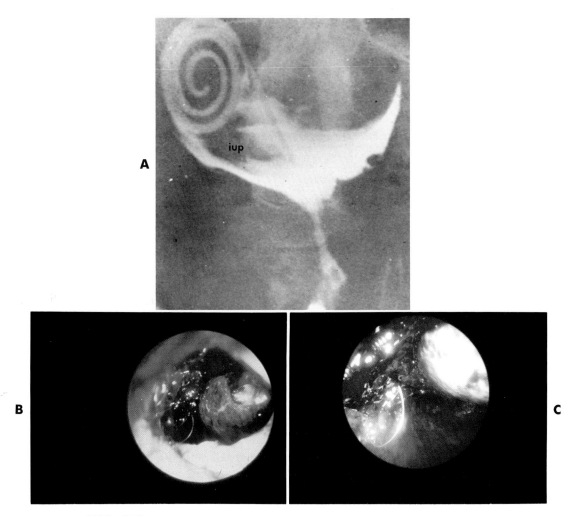

*FIG. 7-9* **A,** HSG shows intrauterine pregnancy (IUP) and IUD pushed to one corner of uterine cavity. **B,** At hysteroscopy, fetal sac is noted and string of IUD is near opposite wall. **C,** Intrauterine pregnancy and IUD. Note string and lower pole of IUD.

## *References*

1. Adel SK, Ghon MA, and Sobrero AG: Hysterographic study of long term effects of intrauterine contraceptive devices, Fertil Steril 22:651, 1971.
2. Alvarez F, Bache V, Fernandez V, et al.: New insights on the mode of action of intrauterine contraceptive devices in women, Fertil Steril 49: 768, 1988.
3. Gentile GP and Siegler AM: The misplaced or missing IUD, Obstet Gynecol Surv 32:627, 1977.
4. Lippes J: Nonmedicated IUDs: history, mechanisms of action and clinical effectiveness. In Zatuchni GI, Daly JA, Sciarra JJ, eds: Gynecology and obstetrics, Philadelphia, 1985, Harper & Row.
5. Millen A, Austin F, and Bernstein GS: Analysis of 100 cases of missing IUD strings, Contraception 18:485, 1978.
6. Rosenblatt R, Zakin D, Stern W, et al.: Uterine perforation and embedding by intrauterine device: evaluation by US and hysterography, Radiology 157:765, 1985.
7. Rowe T and McComb P: Unknown intrauterine devices and infertility, Fertil Steril 47:1038, 1987.
8. Siegler AM and Kemmann EK: Location and removal of misplaced or embedded intrauterine devices by hysteroscopy, J Reprod Med 16:139, 1976.
9. Valle RF: Unpublished data, 1987.
10. Valle RF and Freeman DW: Hysteroscopy in the management of the "lost" intrauterine device, Adv Plann Parent 10:164, 1975.
11. Valle RF, Sciarra JJ, and Freeman DW: Hysteroscopic removal of intrauterine devices with missing filaments, Obstet Gynecol 49:55, 1977.
12. Wagner H: Diagnosis and treatment of complications of intrauterine devices. In van der Pas H, Herendael BJ, Lith DAF, Keith LG, eds: Hysteroscopy, Boston, 1983, MTP Press Limited.
13. Zakin D, Stern WZ, and Rosenblatt R: Perforated and embedded uterine devices, JAMA 247:2144, 1982.
14. Zuanchong F and Yulian H: The experience and management of foreign bodies in the uterine cavity through hysteroscopy. In Symposium on hysteroscopy, Shanghai, Family Planning Association, 1986.

# 8 *Abnormal Uterine Bleeding*

Traditional diagnostic methods to ascertain the cause of abnormal uterine bleeding are anamnesis, physical examination, Papanicolaou smear, and endometrial sampling. Curettage is considered diagnostic and sometimes therapeutic, but the results are sometimes neither informative nor curative.[14] If the location of a submucosal myoma or endometrial polyp has not been identified previously, it is difficult to detect or remove using a curette or forceps. Curettage misses about 25% of the endometrial surface, and in many instances a repeated curettage will fail to disclose an endometrial polyp, a submucous myoma, or an early endometrial adenocarcinoma. Although hysteroscopy is not a substitute for a tissue diagnosis, the endoscopic findings can augment the information available to the gynecologist. Curettage is indicated if the hysteroscopic findings reveal an abnormality; otherwise a random biopsy is probably sufficient.

Modern practitioners of gynecology should not have to justify the importance of hysteroscopy for evaluating the patient who complains of abnormal uterine bleeding or need to emphasize the importance for every hospital to give residents in gynecology and obstetrics departments opportunities to learn the value and technique of diagnostic and therapeutic hysteroscopy.

Using hysteroscopy the gynecologist, while in his/her office, is capable of examining the uterine cavity without causing significant pain for the patient and to safely and accurately assess its architecture. The rate of abnormalities found in patients with abnormal bleeding ranges from 40% to 85%. Hysteroscopy also provides an excellent opportunity to obtain a targeted biopsy of abnormal endometrial areas, and for some patients this procedure represents a method of treatment (Figs. 8-1 and 8-2). Valle[32] wrote that 553 patients who complained of abnormal uterine bleeding had a hysteroscopy before curettage, and 352 (63.3%) showed an abnormality. Among 419 premenopausal patients, 227 (66.1%) had symptoms that could explain their intrauterine abnormalities and findings of 75 (55.9%) of 134 postmenopausal patients were pathologic.

When hysteroscopic findings and biopsy specimens from histologic diagnoses were compared, results in three patients with focal endometrial adenocarcinoma were the same. With a hysteroscopic diagnosis of endometrial hyperplasia, biopsy specimens confirmed the impression in 179 (88.6%) of 202 instances. Adequate tissue was difficult to obtain from submucous myomas seen on hysteroscopy in 70 (87%) of 80 patients.[32] Diffuse endometrial lesions were invariably detected by curettage, but targeted biopsies appeared superior for patients with focal abnormalities. The accuracy of biopsy specimens depends on the visual interpretation of the abnormal area and the adequacy of the endometrial sample.

Gimpelson and Rappold[11] compared the findings of hysteroscopy and curettage in 276 patients. The endoscopic examination revealed more information than the curettage in 44 (18%) women, but curettage was more accurate in 9 instances (3%), and in the remainder of the cases both procedures gave the same result. When 11 patients underwent a dilatation and curettage (D & C) before hysteroscopy, the D & C did not reveal the correct diagnosis in 8 instances. Endometrial polyps were found in 15 women, and leiomyomas were discovered by panoramic hysteroscopy in 13 others. All 28 of these diagnoses were not revealed by the D & C.

Observation of the endometrium may not provide a precise diagnosis, therefore histologic confirmation should be obtained in most instances. If the cavity appears grossly normal, only a random biopsy is suggested. The semirigid biopsy forceps or rigid optical forceps can be used. Although the rigid optical forceps provides better samples of flat lesions, the whole instrument must be withdrawn after the specimen is taken. Care must be taken to retrieve the small specimen from the biopsy forceps. Sometimes the tissue is trapped at the nipple used to occlude the operative channel. Suction curettage is useful if no focal lesion is seen or the endometrium appears diffusely involved. Aspiration curettage is performed with a 4 mm plastic curette.[13] This technique is suitable as an office procedure following hysteroscopy. The advantages of $CO_2$ hysteroscopy (used in combination with suction curettage, if necessary) for the patient and physician are evident.

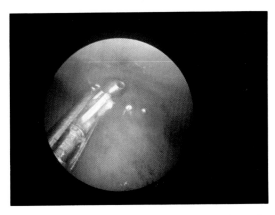

*FIG. 8-1* Endometrial specimen can be taken by directed biopsy under hystero-scopic control.

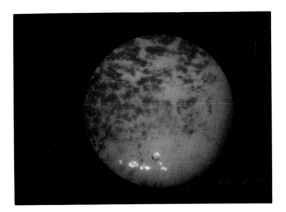

*FIG. 8-2* Endometrium of patient who complained of postmenopausal bleeding. Other than hemorrhagic appearance, no significant abnormalities were found.

## SELECTION OF PATIENTS

When a submucosal lesion is present the hysterogram will show a filling defect, and in many instances this type of abnormality can be diagnosed from an x-ray film. The hysterogram cannot precisely delineate the size or position of the tumor within the uterine cavity, but invariably a normal hysterographic shadow indicates a normal uterine cavity.[7]

Hysteroscopic indications for evaluating abnormal uterine bleeding are similar to those used for endometrial biopsy and curettage. In young women a history, physical examination, and studies to assess ovulation are essential. If the bleeding occurs during ovulatory cycles, hysteroscopy is indicated. Anovulation should be treated with appropriate endocrinologic agents. In perimenopausal and postmenopausal women, a hysteroscopic examination and endometrial sample are indicated before hormonal therapy is prescribed.

## ENDOMETRIAL POLYPS

Endometrial polyps can cause abnormal uterine bleeding, but infertility is infrequent unless the polyps are located in the cornua and occlude the uterotubal ostia, or are large and multiple and interfere with sperm migration or implantation.[34] Polyps that remain after curettage can cause persistent or recurrent, abnormal bleeding. Burnett[2] noted polyps in 121 (9.3%) of 1298 hysterectomy specimens, although half of the patients had a recent curettage. In 42 instances, polyps were the only abnormality found. Word et al.[37] removed 412 uteri immediately after curettage and found 47 benign lesions, including 38 endometrial polyps that had been missed.

### Hysterography

Polyps cause intrauterine defects, seen radiographically as sharply defined borders in various shapes. The defect along the outline of the uterine shadow corresponds to the pedicle of the polyp; it is narrow in the pedunculated ones and broad in the sessile types. An inner radiolucent area can be seen if the polyp is partially coated with medium, but if excessive material is used, the defect is obscured until some fluid is evacuated. A single polyp does not distort the triangular shape of the cavity, but multiple polyps that produce larger defects cause some loss of the uterine outline (Fig. 8-3). Even with large multiple growths, uterine overfilling can mask organic lesions causing misinterpretation. These facts emphasize the need for fluoroscopic control and for fractional instillation of the contrast medium with appropriate spot films to be taken at propitious moments of uterine filling.[29]

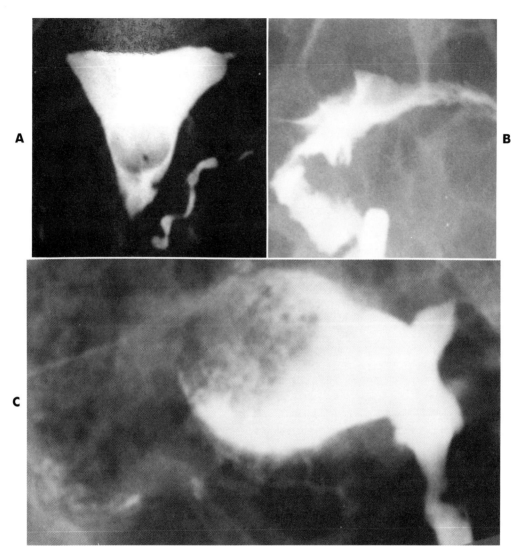

*FIG. 8-3* HSGs show several types of endometrial polyps. **A**, Central filling defect and normal uterine outline was caused by large polyp. **B**, Multiple endometrial polyps distorted shape of uterine cavity. **C**, Large placental polyp was located in right uterine horn. Vascular intravasation is noted.

## Hysteroscopy

If the radiographic examination reveals the suspicion of a polyp, the need for hysteroscopic confirmation and subsequent removal under hysteroscopic control is indicated. Endometrial polyps can be large or small, single or multiple, pedunculated or sessile, and often occur in the fundus or cornu where they are difficult to locate with a curette. They are usually soft, movable, and assume a pink-tan color like the endometrium. The tumors are demarcated clearly from the endometrium and should not be confused with strands of endometrial tissue that seem to hang from the endometrial surface. The size of a polyp can be difficult to measure unless it is compared to a section of the uterine cavity such as the cornu, the uterotubal ostium, or the fundus (Fig. 8-4).

Pedunculated polyps are transected with hysteroscopic scissors and removed with grasping or polyp forceps. Sessile polyps can be curetted, and a repeat hysteroscopic observation can follow to evaluate the effect of therapy. Resectoscopic resection and the Nd:YAG laser have been used but may not be necessary.[6,7]

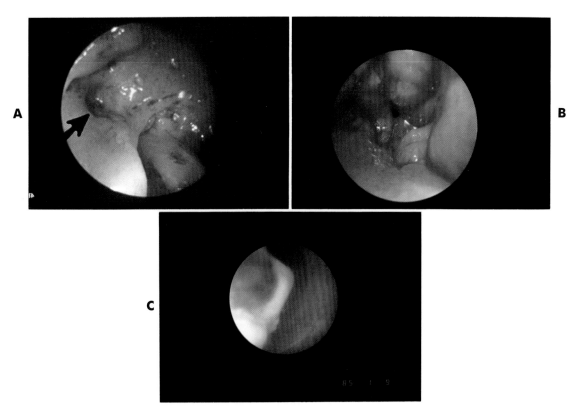

*FIG. 8-4* Endometrial polyps seen in different locations within uterine cavity. **A,** Near uterotubal ostium (*arrow*). **B,** Multiple polyps in left uterine horn. **C,** Placental polyp (see Fig. 8-3, *C*).

## LEIOMYOMA

Uterine myomas are quite common and often asymptomatic, but they can cause abnormal uterine bleeding and infertility. Their detection by pelvic examination is most difficult in the patient who has a normal-sized uterus despite the presence of a significant submucous myoma.

### Hysterography

Submucous and intramural myomas can be seen on hysterography, but serosal or pedunculated types are revealed radiologically only if calcified. Because a submucosal myoma can distort and enlarge the cavity, the hysterogram invariably detects it as contrast material passes around the tumor, often creating a crescentric configuration (Fig. 8-5, A to C).[36] Lower segment or isthmic myomas characteristically cause this region to balloon. In other areas of the cavity submucosal tumors diminish capacity; they can be delineated by small amounts of medium. Other tumors can enlarge the cavity and more than 20 ml of medium is needed to fill it completely. The endometrium that overlies some submucosal tumors is often very thin or necrotic, predisposing the patient to vascular intravasation (Fig. 8-5, D).

The precise relationship of a submucous myoma and the endometrial cavity can be observed by comparative studies of hysterosalpingography, ultrasonography, and magnetic resonance imaging (MRI). Ultrasonography is helpful in documenting the growth of a myomatous uterus over an extended period. Resolution is limited when tumors are adjacent to similar soft tissue densities. With hysterosonography,[26] a rotating ultrasonic transducer protrudes from the front of a stainless steel tube, 8 mm in diameter and 24 cm in length. The uterine cavity is filled with fluid, and during rotation, echo information is collected from the scanning probe and projected to a monitor. Solid, sound absorbing fibroids show sonographic signs of shadowing.

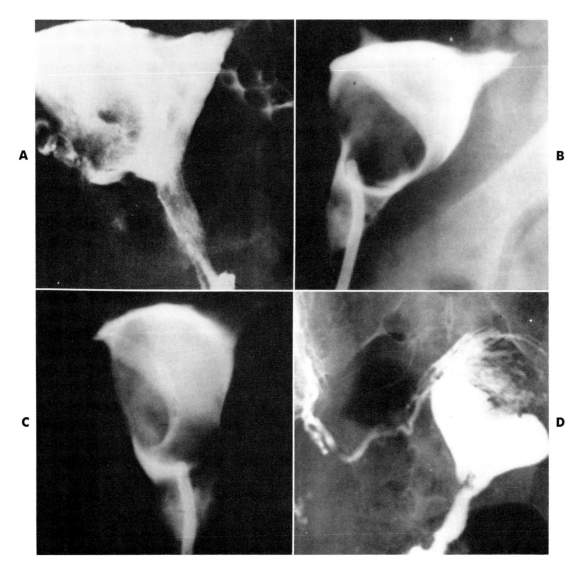

*FIG. 8-5* A, Submucous myoma created filling defect; it also has enlarged and distorted uterine cavity. B, Crescentric formation caused by contrast material passing around myoma. C, Tumor becomes less obvious as additional contrast fluid is added. D, Vascular intravasation occurs near origin of myoma.

## Hysteroscopy

Only a myoma that projects into the endometrial cavity is visible. The endometrium overlying the myoma can be examined with its vascular pattern. The tumor is often lighter in color (almost white) than the surrounding endometrium and is firm when compared to a polyp (Fig. 8-6, *A*). Hysteroscopy allows the examiner to detect, locate, determine if it is pedunculated or sessile, and evaluate its approximate size (Fig. 8-6, *B* and *C*). Porto[27] discovered submucous myomas in 13.4% of his patients evaluated for abnormal bleeding. Sugimoto[30] described the hysteroscopic appearance of various types of submucous myomas, but he did not report removing them hysteroscopically. Valle[32] observed such tumors in 71 (16.2%) of 419 premenopausal patients, and 12 (8.9%) of 134 postmenopausal patients examined had similar abnormalities.

## Hysteroscopic Myomectomy

The traditional treatment for symptomatic submucous myomas has been abdominal myomectomy or hysterectomy. The choice depends on the patient's age, parity, desire to preserve her childbearing capacity and menstruation. Myomas that protrude through the endocervical canal can be removed vaginally, without hysteroscopy. Indications for hysteroscopic myomectomy are abnormal uterine bleeding, pregnancy wastage, and occasionally a submucous tumor has been identified in an infertile patient.[10,35]

Operative techniques include direct hysteroscopic resection using rigid or semirigid hysteroscopic scissors, electrosurgery using cutting loops, a modified urologic resectoscope, and the Nd:YAG laser. Media used for uterine distension include $CO_2$, low-viscosity fluids such as $D_5W$ or $D_5S$, glycine 1.5% using a continuous flow technique, or high viscosity fluids like Hyskon, depending on the experience the gynecologist has using a particular medium and instrument. Every combination of medium and instrument has advantages and disadvantages, but experience is the most important factor. Solutions with electrolytes should not be used with electrosurgery. The operation can be done as an outpatient procedure using general anesthesia.

Deutschmann and Lueken[6] found submucous myomas during hysteroscopy in 67 perimenopausal and postmenopausal patients. Pedunculated myomas were cut and removed, but the number, size, and limitation of the therapeutic interventions were not described. Gallinat[9] limited resection to submucous myomas no larger than 2 cm, and the operation was performed using a special sheath through which rigid instruments such as hook scissors and strong biopsy forceps could be inserted. Valle and Sciarra[33] used semirigid scissors in 34 patients for their method of hysteroscopic resection. Following the procedure, abnormal bleeding ceased in all patients.

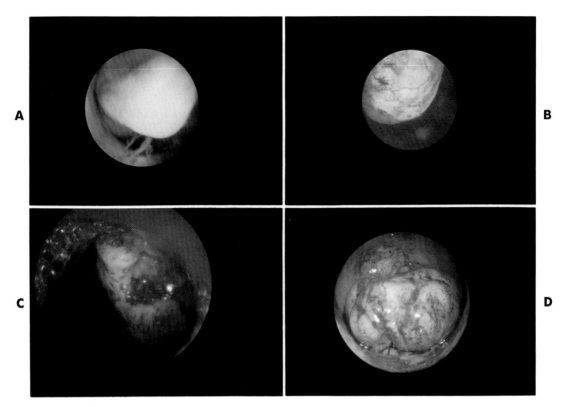

*FIG. 8-6* Variety of submucous myomas. **A,** Large firm tumor obscures uterine fundus and cornua. White color is caused by proximity of light to tumor. **B,** Submucous myoma shows surface vascular pattern. These vessels can rupture, cause bleeding, and predispose patient to vascular intravasation on HSG. **C,** Myoma is in lower uterine segment. **D,** Large submucous sessile myoma occupies entire fundus and extends to both cornu.

### Pedunculated Submucous Myomas

The tumor is first located and then its size and base are determined. If the growth is small (2 cm or less), the pedicle is cut and the myoma can then be pulled through the external os using any of a variety of instruments. Pedicle transection is facilitated by instruments that are sturdy enough to cut thick tissues, but can be easily inserted through the operating channel. Some physicians routinely coagulate the pedicle of the tumor before transection, but experience shows coagulation is not necessary. Once the myoma is removed the myometrium seems to contract and bleeding is prevented. Rigid biopsy forceps fixed to the end of the sheath make it necessary to manipulate the hysteroscope and sheath as a single component, which limits the panoramic view. However, this instrument cuts effectively and expedites the procedure. Large pedunculated myomas require additional cervical dilatation and sometimes morcellation before they can be removed.

Myomas discovered by hysteroscopy can be removed using a large grasping forceps after performing a cervical dilatation using hydrophilic polymer rods or laminaria.[12] With this technique the cervix is dilated to almost 20 mm, occasionally to 27 mm (89 Fr), then a grasping forceps, such as a double-toothed tenaculum, is used to grasp and remove the myoma. This procedure was performed successfully in 83 of 92 patients. In 5 instances, postoperative bleeding required the insertion of a 24 Fr, 30 ml foley catheter as a tamponade. A cerclage was necessary to keep the foley in place.

Pedunculated myomas larger than 3 cm can be systematically shaved with a resectoscope until the pedicle is reached (Fig. 8-7, *A* to *C*). The Nd:YAG laser has been used to resect pedunculated submucous myomas using either the contact or noncontact approach. The pedicle is divided, and the tumor is transcervically removed by grasping it with a sturdy-toothed forceps. Systematic vaporization requires a double-channeled sheath, one channel to irrigate the debris and cloudy medium from the operative field without withdrawing the sheath and hysteroscope, and the other channel is for the quartz laser fiber. Laparoscopic monitoring is used if the dissection is expected to be difficult and myometrial involvement is anticipated.

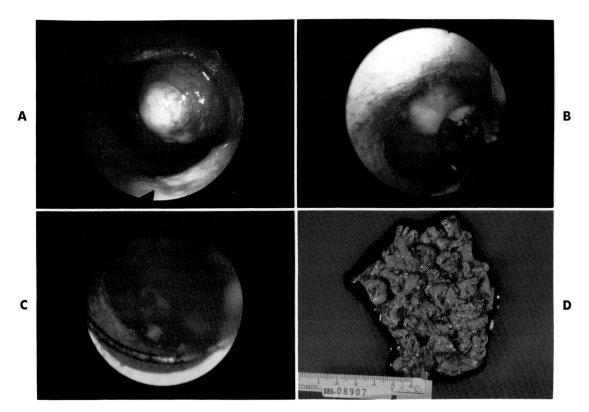

*FIG. 8-7* **A,** Submucous myoma visible along left lateral wall. **B,** Right-angled loop of resectoscope is drawn over surface of tumor to resect. **C,** Completed operation shows normal cavity. **D,** Morcellated specimen from submucous myoma removed under hysteroscopic control using resectoscope. (**C,** Courtesy Franklin D. Loffer, MD.)

### Submucous-intramural Tumors

The surface of these tumors contain prominent vessels in a thin endometrial covering that can be selectively coagulated before the actual dissection begins. When an intramural component exists, partial removal of the tumor may not solve the patient's complaint of abnormal uterine bleeding. The position of the uterotubal ostia must be known to prevent iatrogenic tubal damage. Intracervical injection of 5 to 10 ml of a dilute solution of vasopressin has been advocated to reduce the tendency for bleeding during the myomectomy.

Following cervical dilatation, the resectoscope is inserted, the 90° cutting loop and its electrosurgical attachment are manipulated to familiarize the hysteroscopist with its movement and to allow him/her to check the anatomy and consistency of the tumor. The resection begins with 60 W of cutting current. The electric loop is placed behind the section to be resected and drawn into the insulated sheath toward the objective lens of the hysteroscope. This cutting loop is fragile and the least amount of current should be used. The maneuver should be repeated as many times as necessary to completely remove the myoma. The myoma appears as yellowish-white tissue and should be distinguishable from the myometrium and its pink-tan, coarse, fascicular configuration. Sometimes it is easier to remove the resectoscope and curette the resected fragments that are too large to be removed by irrigation and aspiration. When resected fragments obscure the surgeon's vision, the scope should be removed to allow the tissue to flow out with the medium. The objective end-point of the dissection is to shave the tumor down to the level of the juxtaposed endometrial surface. The tumor fragments can be collected to approximate the size of the original tumor (Fig. 8-7, D).[5,15,22,24]

Although semirigid and rigid scissors are adequate for surgical management of pedunculated myomas, a resectoscope is needed if the myoma is partially embedded in the uterine wall or larger than 4 cm in diameter. Fluids containing electrolytes should not be used for the distending medium. During the gynecologist's training phase this technique should be monitored laparoscopically and done with the assistance of a urologist who has familiarity with these instruments so often used for procedures on the prostate. After the surgeon has decided that the submucous tumor is resectable by hysteroscopy, endotracheal intubation provides the general anesthesia used during laparoscopy. The laser can remove the intracavitary portion of sessile myomas by vaporization. The coagulating effect and controlled delivery of the laser energy are advantages (Fig. 8-8).

Bleeding is controlled during the dissection by the distending medium and postoperatively with either a silastic balloon or an inflated foley catheter. Patients are discharged within 24 hours; the balloon has been removed, and prophylactic antibiotics and a short regimen of conjugated estrogens are prescribed by some surgeons.

Contraindications to hysteroscopic myomectomy are:
1. A large pelvic mass or adnexal tumors
2. A uterine cavity greater than 10 cm in depth
3. A suspicion of malignancy
4. A patient who refuses to accept the possibility of hysterectomy

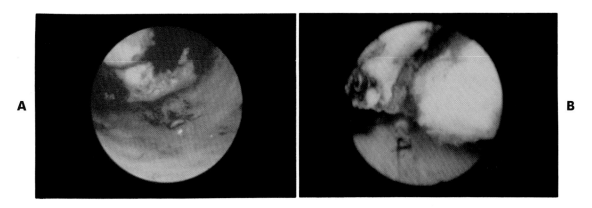

*FIG. 8-8* **A,** Submucous myoma seen near right tubal uterotubal ostium. **B,** Myoma is cut and morcellated by the Nd:YAG laser beam. (Courtesy Jack Lomano, MD.)

## Results

Neuwirth[23] hysteroscopically resected symptomatic submucous myomas in 28 patients and none of them developed any significant postoperative infectious morbidity. Subsequently, 7 patients required a hysterectomy. Among the 17 others, 5 patients became pregnant; 1 delivered vaginally, another had an abdominal delivery, 2 chose elective abortion, and the final patient was in her seventh month of gestation at the time of the report. DeCherney[4] also used the urologic resectoscope for 8 patients to remove submucous myomas; 6 growths were solitary and 2 patients had multiple growths. A 5 ml foley catheter was placed in the uterine cavity for a few hours. Both Neuwirth and DeCherney used high molecular dextran as the distending medium. All of the women left the hospital within 4 to 6 hours postoperatively. Lin et al.[19] removed submucous myomas from 13 patients under hysteroscopic control, but 4 subsequently required a hysterectomy because of adenomyosis or intramural myomas. Lin et al.[18] advocate using a "three contrasts method" with ultrasonography, utilizing a pediatric resectoscope, to monitor transcervical operations for submucous myomas and uterine septa. They claim that it reduces the chance of uterine perforation, especially of the posterior uterine wall, and obviates the need for concomitant laparoscopic monitoring. Their technique included the introduction of about 200 ml NS into the urinary bladder, the infusion of lactated Ringer's solution into the cul-de-sac through the abdominal wall, and 10% dextrose used to distend the uterus. A pediatric urologic resectoscope with a sheath that had an OD of 4.5 mm was used for the operative procedure, and its movements were monitored by ultrasound using an abdominal transducer. Hallez and Perino[16] successfully adapted urologic resection techniques in over 300 cases. The two principles were the use of an endoscope with an electrode to resect or coagulate and a sheath (either 6.3 mm OD or 9 mm OD) that permitted irrigation of the uterine cavity with a continuous nonconductive fluid. The fluid was instilled at about 80 cm water pressure.

A hysteroscopic myomectomy that is successful allows the patient to avoid a laparotomy, a uterine incision, 4 to 5 days of hospitalization, and cesarean delivery should a subsequent pregnancy occur (Table 8-1).

## Perioperative Therapy

Long-acting (GnRH-analogs) gonadotropic releasing hormones can induce hypogonadotropic hypogonadism and estradiol and estrone values fall to castrate levels. These agents reduce the size of some myomas significantly.[3,8] Leuprolide acetate (Lupron) can be administered daily subcutaneously for 4 to 8 weeks preoperatively. The resulting amenorrhea will allow the hemoglobin stores to be replenished. Although preliminary results from these compounds are encouraging, improvements are needed to reduce side effects, simplify administration, and increase the duration of their effectiveness. The use of these drugs could increase the number of hysteroscopic myomectomies performed because they reduce the size of large submucous myomas. Significant shrinkage occurs within 2 months of therapy. No further reduction in the myomas' size occurs after the third month of therapy.

*Table 8-1* Hysteroscopic Myomectomy for Abnormal Uterine Bleeding

| Author | Cases (No.) | Pedunculated | Sessile | Technique | Cured (No.) | Failed (No.) |
|---|---|---|---|---|---|---|
| DeCherney/Polan[5] | 8 | Yes | Yes | Resectoscope/ foley catheter | 8 | |
| Neuwirth[23] | 28 | Yes | Yes | Resectoscope/ silastic balloon | 17 | 11* |
| Lin et al.[18] | 13 | Yes | No | Resectoscope/ rigid scissors | 9 | 4 |
| Valle/Sciarra[33] | 34 | Yes | No | Semirigid scissors | 34 | |
| Goldrath[12] | 92† | Yes | No | Laminaria | 80 | 12‡ |
| Hallez/Perino[16] | 300 | Yes | Yes | Resectoscope | 299 | 1 |
| TOTALS | 475 | | | | 447 | 28 |

All patients treated by resectoscope given Premarin/Provera regimen.
*2 patients lost to follow-up.
†Diagnosis by hysteroscopy; removed by twisting off with tenaculum/forceps.
‡3 patients required laparotomy.

## ADENOMYOSIS

A preoperative diagnosis is difficult because circumscribed adenomyomas are uncommon, and endometrial sampling is not diagnostic. Myometrial hypertrophy causes uterine enlargement, menorrhagia, and dysmenorrhea.

### Hysterography

When diverticula are visible on the hysterogram, they seem to branch out from the uterine cavity. If the glands communicate with the endometrial lining they are outlined by the contrast fluid as it flows into the myometrium (Fig. 8-9, *A*).[28] In some cases a solitary diverticulum is connected to the uterine cavity by a fine channel, but more often perpendicular outpouchings that are multiple and asymmetrically distributed are seen extending from the border of the cavity. Interstitial intravasation results as the contrast fluid enters the glandular channels giving a honeycombed appearance. Sometimes the connections appear as spicular structures that end in small sacs. Areas of adenomyosis that are close to the uterine cavity but do not communicate with it, will not be revealed on the hysterogram.

### Hysteroscopy

The hysteroscopic examination can reveal small, multiple openings (Fig. 8-9, *B,C,D*) along the endometrial surface that explain the outpouching or diverticular pattern seen on the hysterogram.

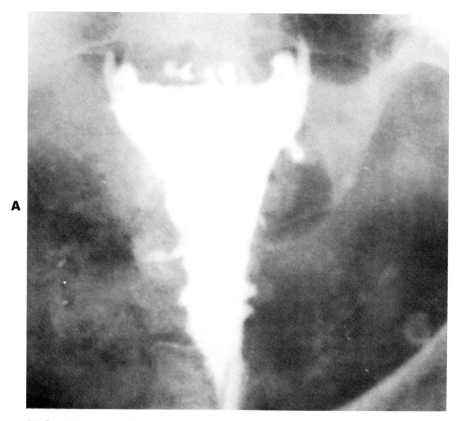

*FIG. 8-9* **A,** Small spicular-like projections seen along the outline of their endometrial cavity are caused by adenomyosis.

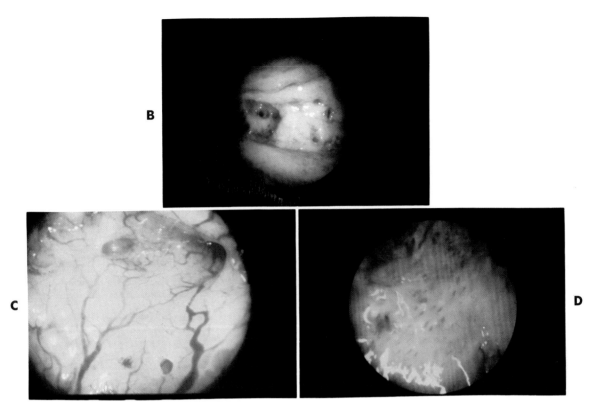

*FIG. 8-9, cont'd* **B,** Hysteroscopic view reveals multiple openings along endometrial surface into which contrast medium extends. **C,** Several endometrial defects shown with increased vascularity on endometrial surface. **D,** View of endometrial surface suggests adenomyosis.

## ENDOMETRIAL HYPERPLASIA
### Hysterography

Although the cavity may appear enlarged with uniform borders that are wavy or scalloped, the hysterogram cannot be relied on to detect this condition. The borders can show decreased opacification when compared to most areas of the uterine shadow. The HSG cannot differentiate cystic hyperplasia from atypical endometrial hyperplasia.

### Hysteroscopy

Polypoid hyperplasia will show as scattered protrusions that are rounded (Fig. 8-10), but cystic hyperplasia exhibits cysts that are blue-gray and translucent. Based on hysteroscopic findings, Mencaglia et al.[21] classified endometrial hyperplasia as low-risk (simple glandular hyperplasia and cystic hyperplasia) or high-risk (adenomatous and atypical hyperplasia). In 78 cases, polypoid hyperplasia, with increased vascularization, was differentiated from hyperplasia with severe morphologic changes. These 8 severe cases were characterized by cerebroid configurations and abnormal vascularization. Of these 8, 6 were confirmed histologically, 1 adenocarcinoma was diagnosed, and the histologic diagnosis for the other patient was decidualization.

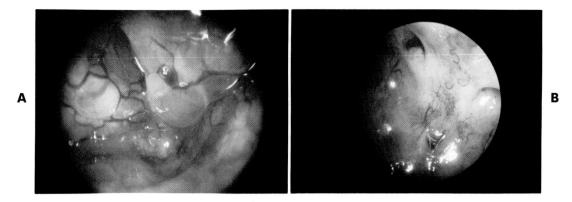

*FIG. 8-10* A, Endometrial surface on biopsy specimen reveals endometrial adenomatous hyperplasia. B, Abnormal vascularization associated with adenomatous
endometrial hyperplasia.

## ENDOMETRIAL CARCINOMA
### Hysterography

Most gynecologists oppose using hysterosalpingography for a patient suspected of having endometrial adenocarcinoma because they believe there is an increased possibility for infection and spread of the disease. Additionally, radiologic signs are not considered to be specific enough. Nevertheless, in some centers[1,25] hysterography has been used as an aid to detect endometrial cancer and to plan the course of treatment (Fig. 8-11). Several medical centers routinely use HSG for the preoperative work-up of patients, and no increase in the risk of intraabdominal or distant metastases has been reported. Experience with HSG and hysteroscopy is similar in 50% of the patients, the medium passes through the tubes. Joelsson[17] found that during HSG, contrast medium was seen less often in the tubes of patients who had developed metastases than in those who had not, and the difference was statistically significant.

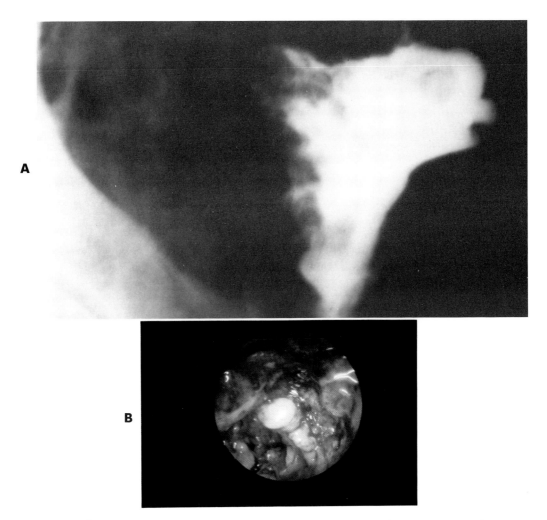

FIG. 8-11 A, Irregular saw-toothed right uterine border in patient who complained of postmenopausal bleeding. Diagnosis of endometrial adenocarcinoma; large, nodular endometrial adenocarcinoma was found. B, Nodular endometrial adenocarcinoma.

## Hysteroscopy

The use of hysteroscopy to examine patients with endometrial carcinoma has been questioned because of the risk of malignant cells spreading through the tubes and into the peritoneal cavity.

Hysteroscopy can confirm the existence, location, and extent of endometrial carcinoma, and a biopsy of a suspicious area is feasible. Sugimoto et al.[31] found 182 cases of endometrial carcinoma during hysteroscopy. The first phase of the examination began without mechanical dilatation of the cervical canal, especially in postmenopausal women. The hysteroscope was applied to the external os, and observations of the cervical canal were made as it was gradually dilated by the distending medium. The hysteroscope was advanced through the internal os toward the fundus and into each cornu. Of the 182 patients with endometrial carcinoma, 167 had circumscribed exophytic growths with polypoid, nodular, or papillary processes often accompanied by ulceration, necrosis and infection (Fig. 8-12) (Table 8-2).

In another series, dextran was used as the hysteroscopic medium for over 100 patients with endometrial carcinoma, and there were no serious complications.[17] Hysteroscopy failed to detect the distal border of the tumor in 3% of the patients, but the malignant growth had reached the cervix by a submucosal extension through the myometrium. Mencaglia et al.[21] detected early endometrial cancer in 7 women under 35 years of age using hysteroscopy. In a later article Mencaglia et al.[20] noted that 59 (90%) of 66 cases classified at hysteroscopy as adenocarcinoma were confirmed on histologic examination. The other 7 women proved to have endometrial adenomatous hyperplasia.

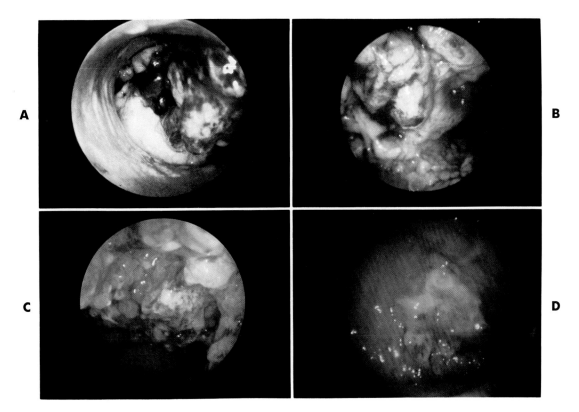

*FIG. 8-12* **A,** Endometrial adenocarcinoma covers entire upper uterine cavity. **B,** Areas of hemorrhage and necrosis in polypoid cancer. **C,** Endometrial adenocarcinoma involves lower uterine segment. **D,** Endometrial cancer localized to cornu.

*Table 8-2* Endometrial Carcinoma: Relationship between Hysteroscopic and Histopathologic Findings

| Hysteroscopic Morphology | Histopathology | | | | |
|---|---|---|---|---|---|
| | Differentiated (Adenocarcinoma) | | | | |
| | Tubular | Adenomatous | Papillary | Undifferentiated | Total |
| Circumscribed | | | | | |
|   Polypoid | 12 | 7 | | | 19 ⎫ |
|   Nodular | 15 | 23 | 4 | | 42 ⎬ 167 |
|   Papillary | | | 71 | | 71 ⎪ |
|   Ulcerated | 4 | 13 | 9 | 9 | 35 ⎭ |
| Diffuse | | | 11 | 4 | 15 |
| TOTAL | 31 | 43 | 95 | 13 | 182 |

From Siegler AM and Lindemann HJ, eds: Hysteroscopy: principles and practice, Philadelphia, 1984, JB Lippincott.

*References*

1. Anderson B, Marchant DJ, Munzenrider JE, et al.: Routine noninvasive hysterography in the evaluation and treatment of endometrial carcinoma, Gynecol Oncol 4:354, 1976.

2. Burnett JE: Hysteroscopy-controlled curettage for endometrial polyps, Obstet Gynecol 24:621, 1964.

3. Coddington CC, Collins RL, Shawker TA, Anderson R, Loriaux DL, and Winkel CA: Long-acting gonadotropin hormone-releasing hormone analog used to treat leiomyomata uteri, Fertil Steril 45:624, 1986.

4. DeCherney AH: Treatment of irregular menstrual bleeding by hysteroscopic resection of submucous myomas and polyps. In Siegler AM and Lindemann HJ, eds: Hysteroscopy: principles and practice, Philadelphia, 1984, JB Lippincott.

5. DeCherney AH and Polan ML: Hysteroscopic management of intrauterine lesions and intractable uterine bleeding, Obstet Gynecol 61: 392, 1983.

6. Deutschmann C and Lueken RP: Hysteroscopic findings in postmenopausal bleeding. In Siegler AM and Lindemann HJ, eds: Hysteroscopy: principles and practice, Philadelphia, 1984, JB Lippincott.

7. Fayez JA, Mutie G, and Schneider PJ: The diagnostic value of hysterosalpingography and hysteroscopy in infertility investigation, Am J Obstet Gynecol 156:558, 1987.

8. Friedman AJ, Barbieri RL, Benacerraf BR, et al.: Treatment of leiomyomata with intranasal or subcutaneous leuprolide, a gonadotropin-releasing agonist, Fertil Steril 48: 560, 1987.

9. Gallinat A: Hysteroscopy as a diagnostic and therapeutic procedure. In Siegler AM and Lindemann HJ, eds: Hysteroscopy: principles and practice, Philadelphia, 1984, JB Lippincott.

10. Garcia CR and Tureck RW: Submucosal leiomyomas and infertility, Fertil Steril 42:16, 1984.

11. Gimpelson RJ and Rappold HO: A comparative study between panoramic hysteroscopy and directed biopsies and dilatation and curettage, Am J Obstet Gynecol 158:489, 1988.

12. Goldrath MH: Vaginal removal of the pedunculated submucous myoma: the use of laminaria, Obstet Gynecol 70:670, 1987.

13. Goldrath MH and Sherman AI: Office hysteroscopy and suction curettage: Can we eliminate the hospital diagnostic dilatation and curettage? Am J Obstet Gynecol 152:2, 1985.

14. Grimes D: Diagnostic dilatation and curettage: A reappraisal, Am J Obstet Gynecol 142:1, 1982.

15. Hallez JP, Netter A, and Cartier R: Methodical intrauterine resection, Am J Obstet Gynecol 156:1080, 1987.

16. Hallez JP and Perino A: Endoscopic intrauterine resection: principles and technique, Acta Europ Fertil 19:17, 1988.

17. Lin BL, Miyamoto N, Aoki R, et al.: Transcervical resection of submucous myomas, Acta Obstet Gynecol Jpn 38:1647, 1986.

18. Joelsson IS: Hysteroscopy for delineating the intrauterine extent of endometrial carcinoma. In Siegler AM and Lindemann HJ, eds: Hysteroscopy: principles and practice, Philadelphia, 1984, JB Lippincott.

19. Lin BL, Iwata Y, Miyamoto N, et al.: Three-contrast method: An ultrasound technique for monitoring transcervical operations, Am J Obstet Gynecol 156:469, 1987.

20. Mencaglia L, Perino A, and Hamou J: Hysteroscopy in perimenopausal and postmenopausal women with abnormal uterine bleeding, J Reprod Med 32:577, 1987.

21. Mencaglia L, Scarselli G, and Tantini C: Hysteroscopic evaluation of endometrial cancer, J Reprod Med 29: 701, 1984.

22. Neuwirth RS: A new technique for and additional experience with hysteroscopic resection of submucous fibroids, Am J Obstet Gynecol 131: 91, 1978.

23. Neuwirth RS: Hysteroscopic management of symptomatic submucous fibroids, Obstet Gynecol 62: 509, 1983.

24. Neuwirth RS and Amin HK: Excision of submucous fibroids with hysteroscopic control, Am J Obstet Gynecol 126:95, 1976.

25. Norman O: Hysterographically visualized radionecrosis following intra-uterine radiation of cancer of the corpus of the uterus, Acta Radiol 37:96, 1952.

26. Popp LW and Lueken RP: Hysterosonography: A new approach for extending endoscopic observations. In Siegler AM and Lindemann HJ, eds: Hysteroscopy: principles and practice, Philadelphia, 1984, JB Lippincott.

27. Porto R: Hystéroscopie. Paris, 1975, Searle of France.

28. Rozin S: Uterosalpingography in gynecology, Springfield, IL, 1965, Charles C Thomas.

29. Siegler AM: Hysterosalpingography, New York, 1974, MEDCOM.

30. Sugimoto O: Diagnostic and therapeutic hysteroscopy, Tokyo, 1978, Igaku-Shoin.

31. Sugimoto O, Ushiroyama T, and Fukuda Y: Diagnostic hysteroscopy for endometrial carcinoma. In Siegler AM and Lindemann HJ, eds: Philadelphia, 1984, JB Lippincott.

32. Valle RF: Hysteroscopic evaluation of patients with abnormal uterine bleeding, Surg Gynecol Obstet 153: 521, 1981.

33. Valle RF and Sciarra JJ: Hysteroscopic removal of submucous leiomyomas (abstract). Presented at Third World Congress and workshop of hysteroscopy, Miami, 1987, American Association of Gynecologic Laparoscopists.

34. Van Bogaert LJ: Clinicopathologic findings in endometrial polyps, Obstet Gynecol 71:771, 1988.

35. Wallach E: Myomectomy: a guide to indications and technique, Contemp Obstet Gynecol 31:74, 1988.

36. Weinstein D, Avaid Y, and Polishuk WZ: Hysterography before and after myomectomy, Am J Obstet Gynecol 129:899, 1977.

37. Word B, Gravlee LC, and Wideman GL: The fallacy of simple uterine curettage, Obstet Gynecol 12:642, 1958.

# 9 *Endometrial Ablation*

Abnormal uterine bleeding, either dysfunctional or associated with benign submucous tumors, may be severe enough to require repeated blood transfusions to correct secondary anemia. Hormonal therapy and repeated curettage may fail to control the excessive bleeding; hysterectomy then becomes the ultimate choice.[6] Successful endometrial ablation should result in amenorrhea or hypomenorrhea. It is appropriate treatment for patients who have blood dyscrasias or medical illnesses and are not good surgical risks. Although a hysterectomy will cure the problem, the peritoneal cavity must be entered, several days of hospitalization are required, the patient will be disabled for several weeks, and there is a potential for morbidity of 20% to 35% of patients. Approximately 600,000 hysterectomies are done in the United States each year, and it has been estimated that 1 in a 1000 of these operations ends in death.[7,10,30]

Many procedures have been developed, as alternatives to hysterectomy, to destroy the endometrium and control excessive bleeding. The intrauterine injection of quinacrine,[31] methylcyanoacrylate,[27] salicylic acid,[20] cytotoxic agents,[3,21] enriched collagen solutions,[24-26] as well as ionizing radiation[22] were used, but none of these techniques proved successful and were not without significant side effects. Droegemueller et al.[8,9] performed cryosurgery to destroy the endometrium by applying a single freeze-thaw cycle of freon after endometrial curettage. All of the patients had a hysterectomy 6 to 8 weeks later and all specimens showed residual endometrium in at least 1 cornu. Of the 16 patients, 10 became amenorrheic before their hysterectomy.

Under hysteroscopic control, using either laser or electrosurgery, it is possible to ablate (volume removal of tissue by vaporization) the endometrium and create severe intrauterine adhesions with subsequent amenorrhea, hypomenorrhea, or at least a normal menstrual flow. To perform this procedure the gynecologist should have experience with the techniques used for operative hysteroscopy and be familiar with the use of lasers and electrosurgery.[2,13,14] In 1986 the Federal Drug Administration approved the Nd:YAG laser procedure for endometrial ablation. The American College of Obstetricians and Gynecologists no longer considers it an experimental procedure.

## SELECTION OF PATIENTS

Most women who have dysfunctional uterine bleeding can be successfully treated with hormones, while those who have benign intrauterine tumors can be cured by removal of the offending submucous tumor. Endometrial ablation should be the treatment of choice if the uterine bleeding is intract-

The authors wish to express their sincere gratitude to Dr. Franklin Loffer for his critical evaluation and suggestions during the writing of this chapter.

148

able or recurrent, if a hysterectomy is medically contraindicated, or if the patient prefers another procedure because of psychological reasons. This operation should not be performed merely to shorten the length of a normal menstrual period. Potential hazards and side effects should be discussed with the patient, including the possibility of hysterectomy in case of complications. A detailed consent form should be signed by the patient.

## PREOPERATIVE PREPARATION

If the patient is of childbearing age, sterilization should be offered because endometrial ablation is not considered a sterilization technique. Since no pregnancies have occurred after 9 years of follow-up in Goldrath's series of over 216 patients,[12] most investigators no longer perform preoperative sterilization. To determine the cause of the bleeding the physician should perform a hysteroscopy in the office. At that time an endometrial sample should be taken to confirm a benign endometrium and rule out the existence of an endometrial polyp or submucous myoma. Often, removal of a submucous tumor, such as a myoma or polyp, will cure the patient and there will be no need to perform an endometrial ablation.

Following appropriate diagnostic procedures, including hematologic studies, it is possible to ablate the endometrial cavity, produce significant adhesions, and destroy the basalis layer. Preoperatively, danazol (Danocrine) 400 mg twice daily for 4 to 6 weeks, is prescribed to thin the endometrium. Alternatively, medroxyprogesterone acetate (Provera) 20 mg to 30 mg daily for 4 to 6 weeks, or megesterol acetate (Megace) 20 mg to 40 mg daily can be used for 1 month. Leuroprolide acetate, a GnRH agonist, can be administered either in daily subcutaneous doses or intramuscularly with depot injections to induce a hypoestrogenic state. Hemoglobin concentrations of 5 to 7 gms/dl will usually increase to 14 gms/dl within 2 months when the patient ingests iron, and the patient will be able to have a unit of autologous blood available before her operation.

## ABLATION
Media

Since Hyskon does not contain electrolytes, an accurate estimate of the amount used must be noted and electrolytes required should be administered intravenously. In addition, this medium tends to develop large bubbles that can obscure the surgeon's vision. This problem can be minimized by repeated flushing. The bubbles tend to migrate anteriorly, so the anterior wall is treated before the posterior and lateral walls. Once they form, the bubbles should be aspirated. By using special hood drapes under the patient's buttocks the fluid withdrawn or that leaks from the uterine cavity can be collected. Baggish and Baltoyannis[3] used Hyskon as the distending medium in 14 patients and a video screen to monitor the operative procedure. In addition, a dual channel sheath allowed simultaneous introduction of the laser fiber and a special polyethylene catheter to aspirate debris.

$CO_2$ has been used as the distending medium during endometrial ablation with the Nd:YAG laser. The intrauterine pressure is preset at 150 mm Hg with an average flowrate of 70 ml/min. Minimal plume is produced below 30 W with the bare quartz fiber. Alternatively, the $CO_2$ can be insufflated directly to the guidelight to blow the smoke from the target area. Since $CO_2$

has no cooling effect, less power is required to produce the desired effect. It is essential that the flowrate of $CO_2$ never exceeds 100 ml/min.

An orthopedic tourniquet wrapped around a plastic, fluid-filled bag can be used to infuse a liquid medium. If two plastic, fluid-filled bags that contain 5% dextrose in NS are connected through Y tubing, and sufficient elevation is given to allow delivery of the fluid at a constant pressure, the uterine cavity can be observed for at least 1 hour. If the patient appears to be absorbing excessive fluid, furosemide (Lasix) can be administered. Another effective method used to maintain a clear field[13] is to have an assistant inject 5% dextrose in NS, contained in 50 ml syringes, during the procedure.

The distending media used most frequently with laser ablation are low viscosity fluids that contain sodium. These can be delivered by mechanical pumps such as the Zimmer apparatus used in arthroscopic surgery. This apparatus injects fluid electronically at preset rates and maintains pressures necessary for adequate uterine distention. The infusion pressure is set at 80 mm Hg and no fluid is instilled unless the pressure falls below the preset value. It is a complicated apparatus for this purpose.

## Sheaths

Some new sheaths have separate channels for the distending media and for ancillary instruments. The sheath described by Baggish[3] has an OD of 8 mm and contains four isolated channels:

1. A 5 mm channel for the hysteroscope
2. Dual 2 mm channels for operative instruments, laser fibers, and aspirating cannulas
3. A 1.5 mm channel for the delivery of distending media

One operating channel can be used to flush the cavity without removing the telescope. Specially designed Luer gaskets are fitted to the operating channels to prevent leakage during introduction of the instruments even if the valves are open. The inflow channel for the distending medium is located on the rotary sleeve and can be maneuvered 360° to provide options for the surgeon. Sheaths with an Albarran bridge can deflect the fiber and direct it to the area to be ablated, particularly to the lateral walls of the cavity.

The endocervical canal is dilated to the size of the sheath to avoid excessive leakage at the external os. If the sheath does not have inflow-outflow channels, the endocervical canal is dilated 1 to 2 mm wider than the sheath to permit egress of debris, mucus, or blood clots. Polyethylene tubing or a ureteral catheter also help clear a cloudy fluid. The bare quartz 0.6 mm fiber is inserted after the spot size has been ascertained.

## Laser

Ablation of the endometrium using Nd:YAG laser energy is a relatively new alternative to hysterectomy to control intractable menorrhagia by photo-coagulation. It involves tissue absorption (uptake) of light energy and converts it into heat. An aiming beam (HeNe laser) is used as a coaxial guidelight with the Nd:YAG laser because, being in the infrared electromagnetic spectrum, it is invisible. The HeNe laser produces a low-power (milliwatts) red light (630 nm) and is used as a guidelight for infrared lasers.[2]

In 1981 Goldrath et al.[12] studied extirpated uteri to assess the effect of lasers, including depth of penetration and their effect on tissue before proceeding with clinical application to 22 patients. To measure the extent of heat transfer, they placed copper thermocouples 1 cm from the endometrial surface and delivered laser energy at 55 W through a 0.6 mm fiber for 5 seconds. The laser fiberoptic was in contact with the tissue specimen perpendicular to the tip of the thermocouple probe. The mean temperature was recorded at 46° C ± 1° C and never exceeded 52° C. During clinical application, the fiberoptic laser beam was in contact with each area of the endometrial surface for a short time. Thermocouples placed on the serosal uterine surface recorded only a mild heating effect. When the Nd:YAG laser was used on the uterine cavity of a hand-held extirpated uterus, no sensation of heat was felt through the uterine wall. In the uterus that is intact there should be greater dissipation of heat because of the cooling effect of circulating blood and the medium used for uterine distention. The endometrium is coagulated, that is, destroyed by heat without physically removing it. This effect brings the temperature to just under 100° C, causing coagulation and subsequent necrosis of tissue. As the temperature of the tissue is raised it passes through several stages: protein denaturation, coagulation, vacuolization, vaporization, and carbonization. The temperature at which these processes occur is not exact and the difference between each stage is not constant. However coagulation and vaporization are the most significant and represent the objective of most laser procedures. As tissue begins to heat above 60° C it begins to desiccate, blanch white, and shrink. Proteins denature and flash boil at 100° C, vaporize, and a smoke plume forms.

When general or spinal anesthesia is used, some physicians recommend a laparoscopic tubal sterilization to avoid the possibility of pregnancy in a severely deformed uterine cavity. Prior to the insertion of the hysteroscope in a 7 to 8 mm sheath, the cervix is dilated to 8 mm to allow egress of the cloudy distending medium during the procedure. Alternatively, the newer sheaths contain a double channel, for inflow and outflow, so the medium can be instilled at a preset flowrate to maintain proper intrauterine pressure and a clear field. The uterine cavity is reinspected to search for submucous tumors.

The Nd:YAG is the laser preferred for endometrial ablation because it can penetrate the juxtaposed myometrium and accompanying vessels 3 to 4 mm, and it can be delivered through a 0.6 mm bare quartz fiber inserted through the operating channel of the hysteroscope. Although thousands of individual fibers are needed to transmit an image, only a single fiber is required to transmit laser light during treatment. The Nd:YAG laser is considered a "cooking" laser and somewhat considered a vaporizing laser. There is better hemostasis but less precision than with the $CO_2$ laser. As a contact coagulation laser, low power (50 W) can be used effectively, and commercial units produce up to 100 W output. Since the inactive endometrium is 1 mm thick, and the myometrium is 20 mm thick, the uterus is a safe organ for this procedure. The Nd:YAG energy beam has a wavelength of 1060 nm and is in the near infrared (invisible) portion of the light spectrum. A HeNe aiming beam is needed to direct and focus the laser to the selected site. This coagulating laser is absorbed by reddish-purple tissue, passes through fluid, and is hemostatic. The surgeon and operating room personnel must wear protective goggles to avoid retinal injury caused by backscattering. A deflector in the ocular of the hysteroscope or operating with a video monitor are safe alternatives.

Endometrial photocoagulation, using the touch or dragging technique, is performed under direct vision with a power output between 50 to 55 W in a continuous wave (cw), a constant steady-state delivery of laser power. Repeated inspection of the endometrial surface will reveal areas that may have been missed. Treated areas change in color from pink, to white, and to brown. If the endometrial surface becomes black, carbonization has occurred, and the laser beam will not penetrate to the planned depth (Fig. 9-1). The topography of the treated area appears as rough channels with the contact in contrast to the smooth surface of the normal endometrium. Care must be taken to avoid uterine perforation at the uterotubal junction, the thinnest area of the myometrium.

Ablation begins by treating the cornua, then the anterior wall, followed by the lateral walls, and last, the posterior wall of the endometrial cavity. The procedure stops at the level of the internal os to avoid a cicatrix at this site. It is difficult to align the fiber perpendicular to the surface of the lower segment so a "dragging" technique is used in this area.

Techniques used for Nd:YAG laser ablation are the blanching (non-touch), dragging (touch), and combination methods. With the dragging technique, endometrial furrows or sulci result as the bare laser fiber touches and indents the endometrium. The visual effects are seen clearly as trench-like lesions and ablated areas are well defined. However, the depth of penetration caused by the front scatter cannot be measured. Unlike the $CO_2$ laser, "you do not see all that you get." Occasionally, bleeding occurs at the completion of the procedure because some superficial myometrial vessels are opened. When the carbon builds up on the fiber, it is removed and gently cleaned with saline.

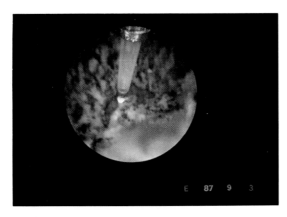

*FIG. 9-1* Dragging (touch) laser technique of anterior endometrial wall performed with the Nd:YAG laser. Some carbonization is noted.

With the blanching technique, the fiber does not touch the endometrial surface (Figs. 9-2 and 9-3). Less debris is accumulated on the bare fiber and there is practically no need to change fibers, since one maintains a working capacity all the time. The fiber is held 1 to 3 mm from the endometrial surface resulting in a blanching effect. Most physicians use a combination of both techniques, utilizing the nontouch methods in the fundal and cornual areas, and the other sections are treated by dragging the fiber across the surface. Sapphire tips also have been used, but in vitro experiments do not clarify that this technique produces the destruction required, even though it does offer the theoretic advantage of simplicity over the bare quartz fiber. The sapphire tip does not tolerate the wattage levels required for endometrial ablation without melting, so only 20 to 30 W are used with this modification. Sapphire tips are excellent for cutting (as in submucous myomectomy or hysteroscopic metroplasty) but not for ablation. Zumwalt et al.[32] wrote that sapphire tips can withstand power levels of only 30 W without melting, and such levels give an inadequate depth of endometrial penetration. Besides, lower wattages require increased operating time.

Lomano[18] compared findings of 17 patients who had endometrial ablation by using the dragging or touch technique with 45 patients who had the procedure done by the blanching or nontouch method. The latter group required less time, less joules of energy, and absorbed less fluid. In addition, 65% of the patients who had laser ablation by blanching developed amenorrhea compared to 12% from the dragging method. It is unsafe to use a sheathed fiber and to instill gas, especially air, into the endometrial cavity. The ablated mucosal surface is predisposed to intravascular intravasation, and excess gas used to cool the fiber can lead to a fatal embolism. Unfortunately several such accidents, although as yet unreported in the literature, have occurred.

The treatment results of more than 216 patients who had excessive uterine bleeding using the Nd:YAG laser have been reported by Goldrath et al.[12] The age of the patients ranged from 12 to 53 years; 130 of them had submucous myomas, and 30 others had adenomyosis. There were 16 patients who had bleeding disorders, 7 of whom were taking Coumadin. Preoperatively, the patients were given danazol (Danocrine) for 30 days to thin the endometrium so there would be less bleeding and greater access to the basalis layer. Laparoscopy was not needed to monitor the procedure and concomitant sterilization was not a requirement. Either general or spinal anesthesia was administered and dextrose and NS were used for uterine distention. About 50 W of continuous energy were employed in a carefully designed technique to avoid missing areas of the endometrium, scarring of the endocervix, or instilling excessive amounts of medium. Marking the junction of the internal os and endocervical canal by circumscribing it before ablation, provided an indication for the lowest margin of treatment. The procedure requires at least 40 to 60 minutes in expert hands, and a good team to monitor the amount of fluid instilled, the amount returned, and to operate the laser machine. Since the anterior uterine wall is the most difficult area within the cavity to treat with the laser, it should be done initially, and then the lateral and posterior surfaces should be done. This sequence is important because debris and bubbles float upward as the procedure progresses and the anterior wall tends to be obscured. To be certain that the entire endometrial surface has been treated, Loffer[15] described using a box pattern of segments with his noncontact (blanching) laser technique. The guiding beam was aimed at the area and then the laser was fired.

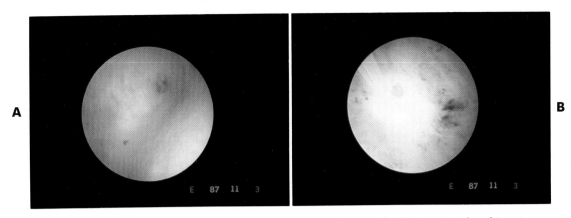

*FIG. 9-2* **A,** Left cornu seen before laser endometrial ablation. **B,** Blanching (non-touch) technique is shown. Note whitish coloration. (Courtesy Jack Lomano, MD.)

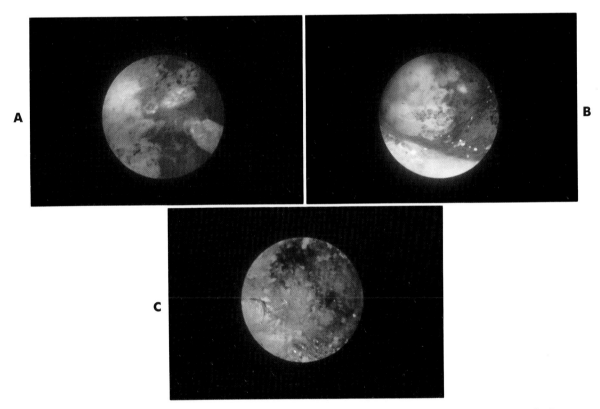

*FIG. 9-3* Stages of endometrial ablation using nontouch or blanching technique. **A,** Laser fiber seen as ablation begins. **B,** One area of endometrium has been destroyed (whitish area). **C,** Aiming beam seen and some carbonization noted. (Courtesy of Franklin D. Loffer, MD.)

Small pieces of detached endometrium must be suctioned because they interfere with the view and reduce the depth of penetration of the laser beam. With the noncontact method, the depth of penetration is less, but it reduces the chance of damage to larger myometrial vessels and decreases the incidence of postoperative bleeding. The power setting is slightly more than with the touch technique. With the noncontact or nontouch technique, the bare fiber is in close proximity to the endometrial surface, the beam is aimed at the specific area, and the coagulation affects a broad area. Although the nontouch blanching technique may be easier to perform, resultant injury is not predictable. The touch technique creates visible defects in the endometrium but three to four times greater damage is done beneath the surface. Both techniques allow in-depth penetration with self-limiting coagulation. The fiber guides continuously move into different areas every few seconds. Because they can inadvertently become coated with debris, backup fiber guides are essential. Tips must be polished if damage occurs. The laser fiber is aimed into one uterine horn and then the other; the fundus and the anterior wall are treated next, followed by the lateral walls, and last, the posterior wall. A series of "boxes" are outlined in each area and the endocervical canal is not treated to avoid any cervical stenosis. Since the tip of the fiber is constantly in view, the chance of uterine perforation is small. There is less chance of injury to large myometrial vessels, the occurrence of postoperative bleeding is reduced, and the degree of intravascular intravasation of the distending fluid is minimized.

Although the $CO_2$ laser is frequently used in gynecologic surgery, it is not appropriate for hysteroscopic procedures.[29] The $CO_2$ laser cannot be used with liquid distending media because the beam is absorbed by water; the Nd:YAG laser will pass through water before it is absorbed. During the evacuation process the HeNe aiming beam cannot be seen clearly because of the smoke plume, which is caused by the vaporization of tissue. The $CO_2$ used as the distending medium is removed, and the uterine cavity collapses. Constant filling and emptying of the uterine cavity, with attention to the limits of the $CO_2$ flowrate, creates significant technical problems.[28] If the $CO_2$ laser could be passed through fibers, it might be applicable for intrauterine surgeries that require resection such as metroplasty or lysis of intrauterine adhesions. Since the $CO_2$ laser acts as a scalpel (cutting) without scattering ("what you get is what you see") and the deeper penetration of the other lasers, its value for endometrial ablation is questionable. If vaporization were to be carried to a greater depth, vessels might be opened and bleeding would result.

The argon laser is also a photocoagulator but much more superficially than the Nd:YAG. It produces a visible blue-green light (488 and 515 nm) and output for medical units is typically about 5 W.

The KTP/532 laser produces a visible green beam that passes through fluid, and it is delivered by a flexible fiber. However, its depth of penetration is half that of the Nd:YAG laser and it does not coagulate as well.

The disadvantages of laser therapy for menorrhagia are:

1. The laser machine is expensive (about $100,000) and a high-technology support system is required in the operating room.
2. The long-term follow-up results are unknown, especially regarding development and detection of occult endometrial adenocarcinoma in pockets of residual endometrium.
3. The surgeon's eyes must be protected from backscatter with a filter or deflector built in the scope's ocular lens or a video camera can be used to monitor the procedure. New microchip endoscopic cameras are now available and the procedure can be viewed on a high-resolution video monitor.
4. The beam produced is capable of causing combustion of drapes, gowns, flammable liquids, or gasses on plastic tubes. To prevent such an occurrence, a nonflammable anesthetic medium should be used and care taken not to expose drapes and other flammable materials near the target tissue area to the beam. Moistening these materials also helps reduce the hazard. Accidental exposure of the laser beam to anything other than the target tissue can cause serious damage. Because of this, background fire extinguishers should be readily available. Reflection of the beam from polished surfaces can occur, therefore eye protection is essential for all personnel.[2,17]

## Electrosurgery for Ablation

A modified urologic resectoscope, 24 Fr (8 mm), with a 30° or 12° lens, but without a drainage valve has been used for endometrial ablation. Electrocoagulation is controlled by a handle mechanism. DeCherney et al.[5] treated 21 patients with intractable uterine bleeding using this instrument. The wire loop was used to excise tissue from around the endometrial cavity and from the intracornual portion of the uterus. The procedure took 15 to 30 minutes. The laser required more time, but 5 patients required the insertion of a balloon catheter to control bleeding.

In a prior study done by DeCherney et al., none of the patients needed a control laparoscopy. The procedures were performed using a local anesthetic with concomitant analgesia and sedation. Of the 21 patients, 18 were still alive after 6 months and had not experienced any further bleeding. The 3 who did not survive died as a result of their primary disease. In 4 of the patients, the use of a general anesthetic was contraindicated, 3 refused to undergo a hysterectomy, and 14 suffered from hemorrhagic disorders. All of the patients required preoperative transfusions. At autopsy the extirpated uteri of 2 patients showed collagen tissue replacement in the endometrium.

Unipolar current with a coagulation setting of 30 to 40 W, and dextran 70/32% w/v (Hyskon) was used because it is nonconductive and provides excellent distention of the uterine cavity. Glycine or 5% dextrose and water can also be used to distend the cavity. Because electrolytes are not contained in these fluids the conduction of electricity is prevented, but it is important to supply the fluids by an intravenous method to prevent water intoxication.

Either coagulation or cutting is used for electrosurgical endometrial ablation. The latter technique removes endometrial tissue as it carves furrows in the uterine cavity. Postoperative bleeding is not uncommon, and compression of the cavity with a 30 ml (24 Fr) foley catheter may be required for a few hours. Less bleeding results with the coagulation technique using either the right-angled loop or the roller ball. The electrosurgical procedure is completed by doing a curettage to remove the coagulated protein.

Electrosurgical units are less expensive than those required for laser therapy. The patient must be grounded. Injury to juxtaposed structures can occur if the instrument penetrates the myometrium, and the depth of penetration is less predictable than with laser energy.[14,21,29] To ablate the endometrium, a ball-end electrode can be used in place of the wire loop. It rolls along the endometrial surface during the coagulation process (Fig. 9-4). Urologists use this device to coagulate areas of the prostate that bleed during a prostatic resection. The ball-end electrode expedites the procedure, permits more complete and uniform treatment of the endometrial surface, and since cutting is not involved, there is less chance for postoperative bleeding and vascular intravasation of media.

Recent innovations in high-frequency electrosurgical units combined with a motor-driven apparatus to monitor the instillation of the liquid distending medium have facilitated electrosurgical ablation.

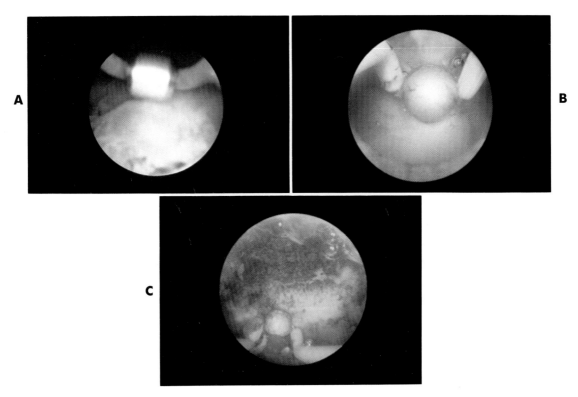

*FIG. 9-4* **A,** Roller ball seen on endometrial surface. **B,** As endometrium is coagu-lated, area turns white. **C,** View of uterine cavity seen after ablation procedure has been completed. (Courtesy Franklin D. Loffer, MD.)

## RESULTS

Patients are usually sent home the day of the procedure, and some women will complain of pelvic pain. A serosanguineous discharge is usually present for about 4 weeks. Postoperatively, the uterus should be sounded at 3 weeks and 8 weeks to prevent a cicatrix at the internal os and development of a hematometra. Most cavities shrink perceptibly and measure 3 to 4 cm in length at the end of 1 month. Hysterograms of 18 patients, obtained 3 to 6 months after the laser procedure, all showed a deformed endometrial cavity characteristic of severe intrauterine adhesions, although in many instances, the proximal portion of the fallopian tubes was opacified.[12] After an electrosurgical ablation the uterine cavity will be small and without intrauterine adhesions.

Endometrial biopsy specimens rarely show endometrial glands. Foreign body giant cells can be seen surrounding carbon particles but there is rarely an inflammatory reaction.[13] Some physicians suggest that danazol (Danocrine) be administered postoperatively for 6 to 8 weeks to allow scar formation before the return of cyclic ovarian activity.[3]

Almost 95% of patients are relieved of their menorrhagia. In the few patients who require a subsequent hysterectomy 6 months or more after ablation, no inflammation or carbon particles is seen.

The objective of therapy should be to cure menorrhagia and not necessarily create amenorrhea. Over 400 cases of endometrial ablation have been reported, and the cumulative results show that 88% of the patients were cured of their menorrhagia (Table 9-1). Intraoperative complications included uterine perforation probably caused by the laser fiber advancing through the myometrium rather than by the laser beam itself. Should a perforation occur, the ablation procedure is stopped, and the patient is observed for symptoms and signs of peritonitis. The urologic application of the Nd:YAG laser to destruct bladder tumors is similar to ablation of the endometrium. The proven safety within the bladder, a much thinner muscular organ than the uterus, demonstrates how minimal the possibility inadvertent uterine perforation is during hysteroscopic use. In a few instances the procedure cannot be completed or fails to correct the menorrhagia. These patients have been successfully retreated in most cases.

Fluid overload can cause facial edema and severe diuresis for 24 to 48 hours. Hyponatremia and hypervolemia can occur in women in whom electrolytes are not used, a phenomenon seen in men after a transurethral resection of the prostate. Prolonged operating time, excessive infusion of irrigating fluid, and opened venous sinuses predispose some patients to fluid overload. These sequelae are potentially serious, and appropriate measures must be taken to avoid them.

Gas, improperly instilled to cool a laser fiber tip, caused an embolism and resulted in death for at least 4 patients. Such information, although undocumented, suggests that improper use of the equipment can lead to fatal consequences.

Perhaps in the future photodynamic therapy can be used to sensitize the endometrium to the dye laser. This technique could simplify and expedite endometrial ablation.[19,23]

Table 9-1 Hysteroscopic Laser Ablation of the Endometrium

| Author | Cases (No.) | Technique | | Duration (Minutes) | Medium Used | Results | | Complications (No.) |
| | | Dragging | Blanching | | | Cure | Failure | |
|---|---|---|---|---|---|---|---|---|
| Goldrath[12] | 216 | Yes | Yes | 30-40 | Low viscosity | 206* | 10 | Bleeding (10) Hypervolemia (2) |
| Daniell[4] | 18 | No | Yes | ? | Low viscosity | 14 | 4 | |
| Loffer[15] | 33† | Yes | Yes | 50-110 | Low viscosity | 31 | 2 | |
| Lomano[18] | 62 | Yes | Yes | 30-60 | Low viscosity | 60 | 2 | |
| Baggish[3] | 14 | Yes | Yes | 40-140 | Hyskon | 13 | 1 | Bleeding (3) Pulmonary edema (1) |
| Gimpelson[11] | 23 | Yes | No | 30-150 | Low viscosity | 22 | 1 | Pulmonary edema (1) Hypokalemia (1) |
| TOTALS | 366 | | | | | 346 (94.5%) | 20 (5.5%) | 18 (4.9%) |

*4 patients retreated, 3 of them cured.
†3 patients followed less than 3 months not included.

## References

1. Babcock WW: Chemical hysterectomy, Am J Obstet Gynecol 7:693, 1924.
2. Baggish MS: Laser endoscopy in obstetrics and gynecology, Clin Obstet Gynecol 26:366, 1983.
3. Baggish MS and Baltoyannis P: New techniques for laser ablation of the endometrium in high-risk patients, Am J Obstet Gynecol 159:287, 1988.
4. Daniell J, Tosh R, and Meisels S: Photodynamic ablation of the endometrium with Nd:YAG laser hysteroscopically as a treatment of menorrhagia, Colp Gynecol Laser Surg 2:43, 1986.
5. DeCherney AF, Diamond MP, Lavy G, et al.: Endometrial ablation for intractable uterine bleeding: Hysteroscopic resection, Obstet Gynecol 70:668, 1987.
6. D'Esopo DA: Hysterectomy when the uterus is grossly normal, Am J Obstet Gynecol 83:113, 1962.
7. Dicker RC, Greenspan JR, Strauss LT, et al.: Complications of abdominal and vaginal hysterectomy among women of the reproductive age in the United States, Am J Obstet Gynecol 144:841, 1982.
8. Droegemueller W, Greer BE, Davis JR, et al.: Cryocoagulation of the endometrium at the uterine cornua, Am J Obstet Gynecol 131:1, 1978.
9. Droegemueller W, Greer BE, and Makowski E: Cryosurgery in patients with dysfunctional uterine bleeding, Obstet Gynecol 38:256, 1971.
10. Easterday CL, Grimes DA, and Riggs JA: Hysterectomy in the United States, Obstet Gynecol 62:203, 1983.
11. Gimpelson RJ: Hysteroscopic Nd:YAG laser ablation of the endometrium, J Reprod Med 38:872, 1988.
12. Goldrath MH: Hysteroscopic laser surgery. In Baggish MS, ed: Basic and advanced laser surgery in gynecology, Norwalk, Conn, 1985, Appleton-Century-Crofts.
13. Goldrath MH, Fuller TA, and Segal S: Laser photovaporization of the endometrium for the treatment of menorrhagia, Am J Obstet Gynecol 140:14, 1981.
14. Jackson R: Basic principles of electrosurgery: A review, Canad J Surg 13:354, 1970.
15. Loffer FD: Hysteroscopic endometrial ablation with Nd:YAG laser using a non-contact technique, Obstet Gynecol 69:679, 1987.
16. Loffer F: Laser ablation of the endometrium. In DeCherney AH, ed: Hysteroscopy, Clin Obstet Gynecol No Am 15:77, 1988.
17. Lomano JM: Photocoagulation of the endometrium with the Nd:YAG laser for the treatment of menorrhagia: a report of ten cases, J Reprod Med 31:148, 1986.
18. Lomano JM: Dragging technique versus blanching technique for endometrial ablation with the Nd:YAG laser in the treatment of chronic menorrhagia, Am J Obstet Gynecol 159:152, 1988.
19. McCaughan JS, Schellhas HF, Lomano JM, et al.: Photodynamic therapy of gynecologic neoplasms after presensitization with hematoporphyrin derivative, Laser Surg Med 5:491, 1985.
20. Richart RM: The use of chemical agents in female sterilization. In Zatuchni GI, Shelton JD, Goldsmith A, Sciarra JJ, eds: Female transcervical sterilization, Hagerstown, Md, 1983, Harper & Row.
21. Rioux JE and Yuzpe AA: Know thy generator! Contemp Obstet Gynecol 6:52, 1975.
22. Rongy AL: Radium therapy in benign uterine bleeding, J Mt. Sinai Hosp 14:569, 1947.
23. Schellhas HF and Schneider DF: Hematoporphyrin derivative photo-radiation therapy applied in gynecology, Colpos Gynecol Laser Surg 2:53, 1986.
24. Schenker JG and Margalioth EG: Intrauterine adhesions: An updated appraisal, Fertil Steril 37:593, 1982.
25. Schenker JG and Polishuk WZ: Regeneration of rabbit endometrium following intrauterine instillation of chemical agents, Gynecol Invest 4:1, 1973.
26. Schenker JG, Nicosia SV, Polishuk WZ, et al.: An in vitro fibroblast-enriched sponge preparation for induction of intrauterine adhesions, Israel J Med Sci 11:849, 1975.

27. Stevenson TC and Taylor DS: The effect of methylcyanoacrylate tissue adhesive on the human fallopian tube and endometrium, Am J Obstet Gynecol 79:1028, 1972.

28. Tadir Y, Raif J, Dagan J, et al.: Hysteroscope for $CO_2$ laser application, Laser Surg Med 4:153, 1984.

29. Taylor KW and Desmond J: Electrical hazards in the operating room with special reference to electrosurgery, Canad J Surg 13:362, 1970.

30. Wingo PA, Huezo CM, Rubin GL, et al.: The mortality risk associated with hysterectomy, Am J Obstet Gynecol 152:803, 1985.

31. Zipper J, Medel M, Pastene I, et al.: Intrauterine instillation of chemical cytotoxic agents for tubal sterilization and treatment of functional metrorrhagias, Int J Fertil 14:289, 1969.

32. Zumwalt T, Wesseler T, and Joffe SN: A comparison of artificial sapphire tip with quartz tip in in vitro endometrial ablation, Colpos Gynecol Laser Surg 2:47, 1986.

# 10 *Tubal Cannulation*

Gardner[13] in 1856 in his text, *The Causes and Curative Treatment of Sterility,* described and illustrated passing a probe through the intramural segment (Fig. 10-1). A series of graduated instruments were used to overcome tubal strictures, but there was no direct observation of the maneuvers. This method had apparently been previously attempted by W. Tyler Smith in 1849.

In addition to allowing access to the uterotubal ostia for the purpose of sterilization, cannulating tubes could be used therapeutically, to overcome tubal obstruction,[8,23] for tubal insemination,[4,14] to transfer gametes,[18,19] and to study tubal function.[21]

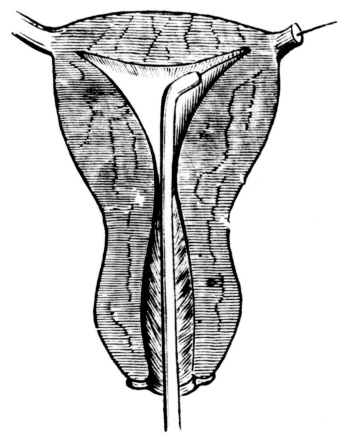

*FIG. 10-1* Wire guided through intramural segment. (From Gardner AK: The causes and curative treatment of sterility with a preliminary statement of the physiology of generation, New York, 1856, DeWitt & Davenport.

## TUBAL ANATOMY

It is appropriate to briefly review the anatomy of the proximal tubal segment; the location for these intratubal maneuvers. The fallopian tubes are paired organs about 10 cm long (with variations in length from 7 to 14 cm) and are enclosed in the mesosalpingeal borders of the broad ligament. They are lined with a specialized mucous membrane and emerge from the uterine cornua at the junction of the corpus and fundus. This anatomic connection allows the nonoperative tubal patency tests to be done, but it also is a potential route for ascending pelvic infections.

## Intramural Segment
### Interstitial Portion

This section, lying within the myometrium, measures slightly less than 2 cm in length and varies from 0.2 to 0.4 mm in diameter. Lisa et al.[16] examined 300 extirpated uteri and found 33 instances of tubal polyps in this tubal segment, which were always endometrial in nature (Fig. 10-2). No anatomic uterotubal sphincter was demonstrated. A report on 100 intramural segments taken from freshly extirpated uteri disclosed that 69 uteri were tortuous, 23 uteri were straight, and 8 uteri appeared to be curved; their lengths varied from 1 to 3.5 cm. The intramural portion, extending about 2 cm from the cornu, includes the pretubal bulge (Fig. 10-3).[24]

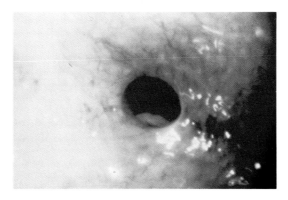

*FIG. 10-2* Small polyp seen in intramural segment.

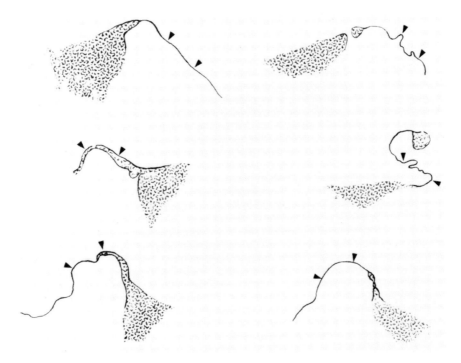

*FIG. 10-3* Schematic representation illustrates various shapes of the intramural segment. Arrow heads are 1 cm and 2 cm from cornua.

*Pretubal Bulge*

There is an ampulla-like dilatation of the intramural segment just proximal to its termination. This area, shaped like a small triangle, has its base toward the uterus, its apex toward the tubal isthmus, and has straight or convex side walls (Fig. 10-4). It is this area that can be seen clearly during hysteroscopy (Fig. 10-5). An interruption in tubal continuity is often present preceding the bulge, since the shadow just lateral to the constriction is intramural.

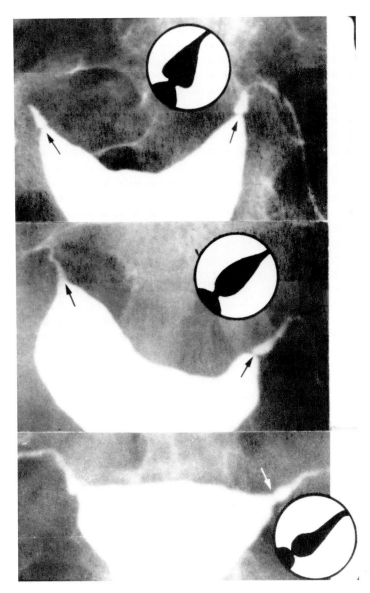

*FIG. 10-4* HSGs and insets show three forms of pretubal bulges.

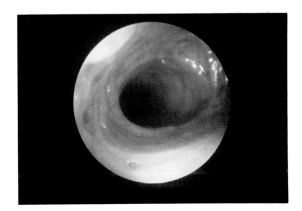

*FIG. 10-5* Proximal part of tube is visible.

The anatomic basis for this radiologic picture is the fold at the transition between the endometrium and endosalpinx (Fig. 10-6). The "membrane" is often seen at the uterotubal ostium during hysteroscopy (Fig. 10-7). Its absence is not related to the stage of the cycle and it appears to be of minimal clinical significance.

In an analysis of 1000 salpingograms, the bulge appeared bilaterally in 33% and unilaterally in 23.5%, the dark line usually occurred at the base of the triangle and separated it from the intramural segment. Three shapes of bulges can be seen radiologically.[22] Usually the continuity of the uterotubal junction is not interrupted, but a perceptible annular constriction is seen when the lateral shadow exists in various forms. In other instances, a small shadow cuts obliquely through the apex of the uterine horn, and the lateral portion appears as a small equilateral triangle or an elongated funnel with relatively distinct corners. Sometimes the base is rounded and the bulge is club-shaped. The third variation has a second interruption in the isthmus near the bulge which is caused by tubal contractions. These configurations are not consistent on successive roentgenograms nor do they necessarily reappear in their initial form in repeat HSGs.

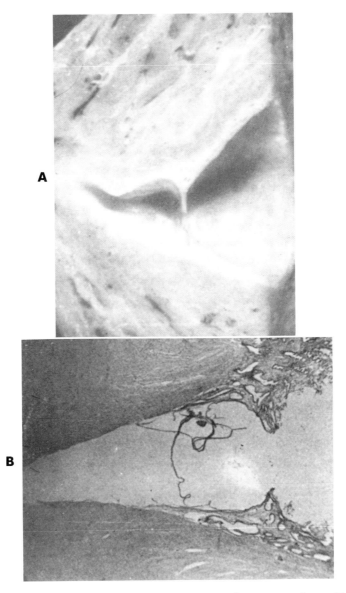

*FIG. 10-6* **A,** Cut surface of intramural segment shows "membrane" between endometrium and endosalpinx. **B,** Histologic section reveals endometrium and endosalpinx ( × 60).

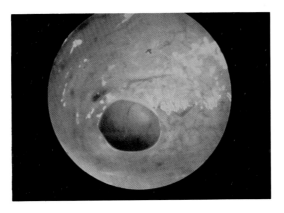

*FIG. 10-7* Thin membrane separates endometrium from endosalpinx seen hysteroscopically.

## ISTHMUS

The twists and turns of the tubal isthmus are usually more illusory than real, depending on its position in relation to the film. It is not possible to radiographically measure the length of this portion precisely. The isthmus is the narrowest extrauterine tubal segment, its lumen is about 2 mm wide and is 2 to 3 cm long. The muscular layers of the isthmus are the thickest and most clearly defined of the major tubal segments. When the lumen is not opacified but the ampulla appears filled, the tubal isthmus is assumed to be patent.

## INDICATIONS FOR TUBAL CANNULATION
### Proximal Tubal Obstruction

Cornual spasm causing pseudoocclusion is always a possibility when the tubes fail to opacify on the HSG or do not fill during the laparoscopy.[1,6,26] Careful technique in the performance and studied interpretation of these tests will help to minimize this cause of proximal tubal obstruction.

#### Hysterosalpingography

The initial test to search for proximal tubal obstruction is the HSG. It is important for the gynecologist and radiologist to be aware of the type and amount of contrast material that is used and when to end the examination. Increasing abdominal pain indicates that the uterine cavity has been filled to its capacity, and failure to see tubal opacification on the fluoroscopic screen denotes proximal obstruction. In almost all instances of a properly performed HSG, the cornua are pointed, the intramural segment is filled and often a pretubal bulge is seen. Causes of proximal tubal disease detected radiographically include salpingitis isthmica nodosa, endometriosis, tubal polyps, and tuberculous salpingitis. Multiple isthmic diverticuli can be seen with either salpingitis isthmica nodosa or severe endometriosis affecting the proximal tubal segment. Such findings are contraindications to attempted tubal catheterization.

#### Laparoscopy

Having made a presumptive diagnosis based on the history, clinical examination, and the hysterosalpingogram, the next procedure is to view the pelvis endoscopically and examine the tubes and ovaries that are not visible roentgenographically. The shape and consistency of the isthmus should be observed. Nodularity and firmness can corroborate the diagnosis of salpingitis isthmica nodosa, whereas a grossly normal tube would indicate probable luminal occlusion caused by fibrosis. Chromopertubation is essential and should be attempted several times, occasionally changing cannulas. Spasm or pseudoocclusion must always be considered for these patients and repeated attempts at chromopertubation should be carried out. In addition to looking at the proximal segment to ascertain the cause and type of obstruction, laparoscopy allows evaluation of the rest of the pelvis.

### Transcervical Tubal Catheterization

The corroboration and subsequent treatment of proximal tubal obstruction varies with the cause of the obstruction and often requires an operative procedure to remove the diseased portions of the fallopian tube. In about 10% to 15% of the patients who have had resections to the proximal tubal segment in preparation for a tubotubal anastomosis, no histologic evidence of occlusion was seen in the excised tissue.[12] With such evidence and the report of the occurrence of tubal "plugs,"[23] transcervical catheterization should be attempted prior to microsurgical anastomosis to dislodge such material and to break up mild intraluminal adhesions.

Daly et al.[7] found adhesions covering the uterotubal ostia that were not detected by HSG. In 3 patients these meshlike adhesions were removed with a hysteroscopic biopsy forceps, and the patients conceived within 3 months. Dolff[11] described salpingocatheterization of the uterotubal segment with a No. 3 Charriere ureteral catheter. The inability to induce contractions at the tubal angle by catheterization indicated fibrosis. Mencaglia et al.[17] performed transcervical salpingoscopy in 228 infertile patients and 41 abnormalities were seen in the right ostium and 37 in the left. Fifty-five (70%) were called atretic ostia. Cornual adhesions and polyps accounted for 15 (19%), and almost all of the polyps were removed hysteroscopically. Confino et al.[5] described using a transcervical balloon for dilatation and recanalization of a proximally obstructed tube.

The catheter and guidewire were advanced through the operating channel of the hysteroscope. After the guidewire was inserted into the interstitial part of the tube, the balloon was inflated with water-soluble opaque material. The guidewire was removed, the contrast media was instilled, and a salpingogram showed a patent tube. This ostial salpingography was done under laparoscopic control. Deaton et al.[9] recanalized the tubes in 7 of 10 patients who had proximal tubal obstruction using a urologic catheter and a flexible guidewire. Laparoscopic control disclosed 1 perforation without sequelae. Transvaginal fluoroscopic recanalization of a proximally occluded oviduct was reported by Platia and Krudy[20] who used a 0.7 mm guidewire passed into a No. 3 Fr end-hole polyethylene catheter. Patency was established in 1 tube and the patient became pregnant. This type of procedure could be adapted to a hysteroscopic approach.

Selective transcervical catheterization of the fallopian tubes using a modified angiographic technique and fluoroscopic guidance can be used to diagnose and treat selected cases of proximal tubal obstruction.[10,25] The first step of a transcervical catheterization is ostial salpingography. The contrast medium is injected into the uterotubal ostium, and the injection should be stopped when there is absence of tubal filling, vascular intravasation occurs, there is increased abdominal pain, or the medium flows back into the uterine cavity. If ostial salpingography fails to opacify the tube, tubal canalization is the next step. A No. 3 Fr catheter is used and a guidewire 0.046 cm (0.5 mm) is passed through it. With this coaxial catheter set, 27 of 28 proximally obstructed tubes were opened under fluoroscopic guidance with only 1 minor complication (Fig. 10-8).[25]

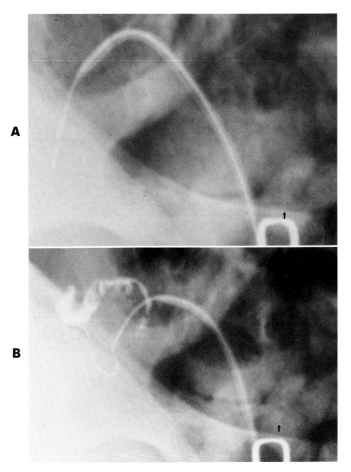

*FIG. 10-8* Technique for transcervical tubal cannulation (*t*, tenaculum). **A**, Catheter is placed in intramural segment. **B**, Contrast material has entered fallopian tube.

*Transfer of Gametes and Embryos*

In 1984 Asch et al.[2] reported a pregnancy following a procedure defined as gamete intrafallopian tube transfer (GIFT) that consisted of depositing the ovum and spermatozoa into the fallopian tube. They performed subsequent procedures by doing either a laparotomy or laparoscopy. $CO_2$ was used for pneumoperitoneum.

Several methods of tubal transfer of gametes during hysteroscopy are possible using $CO_2$ as the distending medium. These include intratubal insemination of washed sperm, the transfer of washed sperm and oocytes, and the transfer of 2-4 cell stage embryos. Unless the fallopian tube, as a result of laparoscopic chromopertubation, appears grossly normal and patent, a tubal pregnancy can result from hysteroscopic transfers of gametes or embryos.

The fundamental characteristics of a catheter used for such a transfer include a width between 0.8 to 1 mm and proper rigidity to allow nontraumatic tubal catheterization. Single and double catheters can be used. A double catheter has already been developed for laparoscopic GIFT. The outer catheter, 1 mm OD, cannulates the uterotubal ostium and the inner catheter, 0.7 mm OD, is loaded with gametes and inserted into the outer catheter. One potential problem is the possibility the intrauterine pressure might push the gametes through the tube into the peritoneal cavity. Based on similar results from laparoscopic GIFT and laparotomy,[3] the $CO_2$ used during hysteroscopy should not cause concern. During hysteroscopic GIFT, intrauterine pressure is maintained at 40 to 50 mm Hg. As soon as the catheter enters the uterotubal ostium, the flow of $CO_2$ is stopped. The method used for loading the catheter is similar to the one used for laparoscopic GIFT. Sperm are prepared following standard washing and swim-up procedures. Intratubal insemination is performed with 100,000 to 300,000 capacitated spermatozoa in 50 to 70 $\mu$l of buffer. One to five oocytes are inserted into the catheter (Figs. 10-9 to 10-11). Only 1 tube is catheterized because deposited gametes would be pushed into the peritoneal cavity during catheterization of the second tubal ostium.

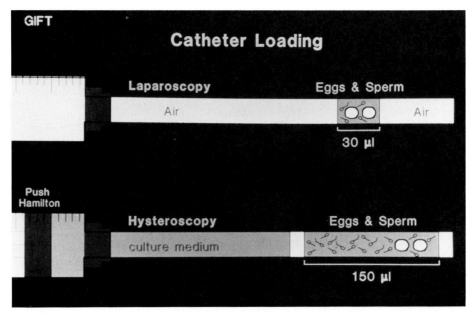

*FIG. 10-9* Methods for loading catheter for hysteroscopic and laparoscopic GIFT procedure.

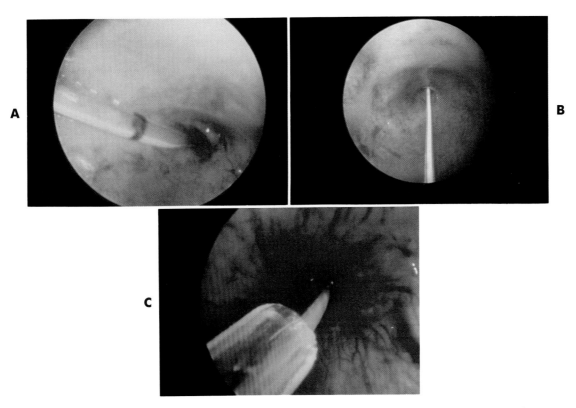

*FIG. 10-10*  **A,** Loaded catheter placed in intramural segment. **B,** Another catheter used for transfer of gametes. **C,** Double-lumen catheter is shown.

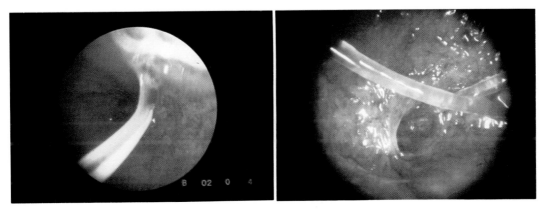

*FIG. 10-11* Technical problems can prevent proper alignment of catheter and uterotubal ostium.

Studies on 25 patients who had normal fallopian tubes revealed that:
1. The injection pressure in the syringe can push 100 $\mu$l of methylene blue to the fimbriated end of the tube.
2. The catheter should be loaded with no more than 70 $\mu$l.
3. It is important to fill the empty part of the catheter and syringe with liquid because the intrauterine pressure tends to push the oocytes and the spermatozoa back into the catheter.

Gubbini et al.[14] reported 80 intratubal inseminations under hysteroscopic guidance followed by 3 pregnancies. Colacurci et al.[4] described results from 51 hysteroscopic intratubal inseminations compared to a control group of 54 intraperitoneal inseminations; five pregnancies resulted from intraperitoneal inseminations but only 2 were in the hysteroscopic group. In another series of 79 hysteroscopic intratubal inseminations, 2 pregnancies resulted.[4] Other investigators have described similar outcomes.[18,19,26,27]

Ultrasound-guided–tubal-embryo-transfer (UG-TET) was described by Jansen et al.[15] and a pregnancy was reported. A No. 3 Fr teflon catheter tapered to No. 2 Fr was inserted into a sheath (No. 5 Fr) and then passed 3 cm beyond the outer sheath and inserted into the uterotubal ostium (Fig. 10-12).

Tubal catheterization under hysteroscopic control has several potential uses and constitutes an interesting area for research in reproduction.

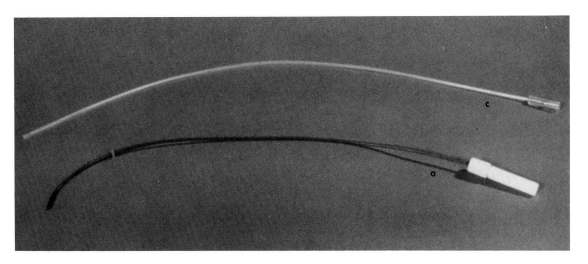

*FIG. 10-12* Jansen catheter (*c*) is shown with obturator (*o*).

*References*

1. Alper MM, Garner PR, and Spence JEH: Hysocine butylbromide to relieve uterotubal obstruction at hysterosalpingography, Brit J Radiol 58:915, 1985.
2. Asch RH, Ellsworth LR, and Balmaceda JP: Pregnancy after trans-laparoscopic gamete intrafallopian tube transfer (GIFT), Lancet 2:1034, 1984.
3. Asch RH, Balmaceda JP, Cittadini E, et al.: GIFT: international cooperative study. The first 800 cases. Ann NY Acad Sci 541:722, 1988.
4. Colacurci N, DePlacido G, Perrone D, et al.: La inseminazione tubarica per via endoscopica. In Cittadini E, Scarselli G, Mencaglia L, et al., eds: Isteroscopia operativa e laser chirurgia in ginecologia, Rome, 1988, CIC Edizioni Internazional.
5. Confino E, Friberg J, and Gleicher N: Transcervical balloon tuboplasty, Fertil Steril 46:963, 1986.
6. Cooper JM, Rigberg HS, Houck R, et al.: Incidence, significance and remission of tubal spasm during attempted hysteroscopic tubal sterilization, J Reprod Med 30:39, 1985.
7. Daly DC, Soto-Albors CE, and Aversa MA: Hysteroscopic detection and treatment of adhesions at the tubal ostium/uterine junction in infertile patients, Fertil Steril 46:138, 1986.
8. Daniell JF and Miller W: Hysteroscopic correction of cornual occlusion with resultant term pregnancy, Fertil Steril 48:490, 1987.
9. Deaton JL, Gibson M, Riddick DH, et al.: Diagnosis and treatment of cornual obstruction using a flexible tip guidewire, Abstract, Am Fertil Soc Prog Suppl 102:35, 1988.
10. DeCherney AH: Anything you can do I can do better . . . or differently, Fertil Steril 48:374, 1987.
11. Dolff M: Carbon dioxide hysteroscopy before tubal microsurgery. In Siegler AM and Lindemann HJ, eds: Hysteroscopy: principles and practice, Philadelphia, 1984, JB Lippincott.
12. Fortier KJ and Haney AF: The pathologic spectrum of uterotubal junction obstruction, Obstet Gynecol 65:93, 1985.
13. Gardner AK: The causes and curative treatment of sterility with a preliminary statement of the physiology of generation, New York, 1856, DeWitt & Davenport.
14. Gubbini G, Tabanelli C, Guerra B, et al.: Inseminazione intratubarica, Fisiopat Rip 6:80, 1988.
15. Jansen RPS, Anderson JC, Sutherland PD: Nonoperative embryo transfer to the fallopian tube, N Engl J Med 319:288, 1988.
16. Lisa JR, Gioia JD, and Rubin IC: Observation of the interstitial portion of the fallopian tube, Surg Gynecol Obstet 99:159, 1954.
17. Mencaglia L, Hamou J, Perino A, et al.: Transcervical and retrograde salpingoscopy; evaluation of the fallopian tube in infertile patients. In Siegler AM and Ansari AH, eds: The fallopian tube: basic studies and clinical contributions, New York, 1986, Futura.
18. Miyazaki K, Fukuda Y, Tsiji Y, et al.: Gamete intrafallopian tube transfer under hysteroscopic control, Presented at XII World Congress of Obstet Gynecol, Free communications, 1988, Rio de Janeiro.
19. Perino A, Venezia R, Catinella E, et al.: Trasferimento intratubarico di gameti sotto controllo isteroscopico. In Cittadini E, Scarselli G, Mencaglia L, et al., eds: Isteroscopia operativa e laser chirurgia in ginecologia, Rome, 1988, CIC Edizioni Internazional.
20. Platia MP and Krudy AG: Transvaginal fluoroscopic recanalization of a proximally occluded oviduct, Fertil Steril 44:704, 1985.
21. Quinones GR, Alvarado DA, and Aznar RR: Tubal catheterization applications of a new technique, Am J Obstet Gynecol 114:674, 1974.
22. Siegler AM: Hysterosalpingography, 2nd ed, New York, 1974, Medcom Press.
23. Sulak PJ, Letterie GS, Hayslip CC, Coddington CC, and Klein TA: Hysteroscopic cannulation and lavage in the treatment of proximal tubal occlusion, Fertil Steril 48:493, 1987.

24. Sweeney WJ: The interstitial portion of the uterine tube: its gross anatomy, course, and length, Obstet Gynecol 19:3, 1963.
25. Thurmond AS, Novy M, Uchida BT, et al.: Fallopian tube obstruction: Selective salpingography and recanalization, Radiology 163:511, 1987.
26. World Health Organization: A new hysterographic approach to the evaluation of tubal spasm and spasmolytic agents, Fertil Steril 39:105, 1983.
27. Wurfel W, Krushmann G, Rotenoncher M, et al.: Schwangershaft nach intratubaren Gameten Transfer per Hysteroscopien, Geburtsh Frauenhlk 48:401, 1988.

# 11 *Hysteroscopic Sterilization*

For more than a century physicians have searched for a method to occlude the fallopian tubes at their uterotubal ostia. The width of the ostium in the intramural segment is about 1 mm ± 0.5 mm, 2 cm in length, and the lumen is linned with a single layer of low columnar cells. The surrounding three-layered muscular wall is the thickest area of the fallopian tube and although visual evidence of contractions has been seen during hysteroscopic examinations, no sphincter has been identified. Technical advances in endoscopic methods and an increasing demand for a safer sterilization technique encouraged investigators to use hysteroscopy to obstruct the interstitial tubal segment.

The potential advantages of a transcervical operation are the elimination of general anesthesia, the avoidance of an abdominal incision, and the potential for intraabdominal adhesions. Access to the tubal ostia for sterilization can be by a direct or indirect transcervical approach. The techniques are in two categories:

1. Destructive operations where the intramural segment is destroyed by electrosurgery or sclerosing agents
2. Mechanical occlusion of the uterotubal ostia using plugs or devices

In 1849 Froriep[11] infused a solution of silver nitrate into the uterine cavity to occlude the interstitial tubal segment. Kocks,[16] in 1878, reported a transuterine sterilization by cauterizing the ostia. Techniques using specially designed probes[8,9,14] and balloons, without the benefit of direct observation have been described, but tubal occlusion and sterilization were unpredictable and occurred in less than 80% of the patients.

## Electrosurgery

The endoscopic or direct visual approach to the tubal ostia for sterilization purposes was initially suggested by von Mikulicz-Radecki and Freund in 1927.[20] They cited the need to destroy the endosalpinx and part of the juxtaposed myometrium to prevent regeneration or recanalization after coagulation of the intramural segments in experimental animals. A few of these operations were performed on women but a hysterectomy followed soon after to study the effects on the tissues. Schroeder[29] described the results of hysteroscopic tubal sterilization using electrocoagulation in 2 women which he followed by HSGs 2 weeks postoperatively. Both patients showed postoperative tubal patency and they were subsequently sterilized by laparotomy. Norment et al.[22] described tubal sterilization by fulguration of the cornual ostia under hysteroscopic control, but they never disclosed the number of patients or the results (Table 11-1).

*Table 11-1* Historical Development of Hysteroscopic Tubal Sterilization with Electrosurgery

| Author | Year | Contribution |
|---|---|---|
| von Mickulicz-Radecki/ Freund[20] | 1927 | Fulguration experiments on animals Human studies; immediate hysterectomy |
| Schroeder[29] | 1934 | Fulguration on 2 patients; postoperative HSG showed patency; laparotomy sterilization |
| Norment[22] | 1956 | Fulguration, but number of patients and outcome not stated |
| Sugimoto[31] | 1974 | 38 patients, outcome unknown |
| Lindemann/Mohr[18] | 1974 | 124 patients; HSG 12 weeks postoperative; at least 1 tubal patency in 33 women |
| Neuwirth et al.[21] | 1975 | 93 patients; HSG followed sterilization; tubal patency in 20% |
| Quinones et al.[24] | 1976 | HSG in 552 patients; tubal patency in 17%; pregnancy in 6 patients |
| Darabi et al.[5] | 1977 | Collaborative study of 773 patients; HSG in 524; tubal patency in 33%; pregnancy in 70 patients |

In the 1970s many studies were published about advantages of electro-coagulation of the uterotubal ostia.* Hysteroscopic tubal sterilization (HTS) with electrosurgery required the following:

1. A skilled hysteroscopist who could consistently locate the ostia
2. An end-point objective to know when the procedure was complete
3. Special probes to safely enter the uterotubal ostia without penetrating the myometrium
4. Careful application of the electrosurgical energy, the wattage and length of time needed to complete the procedure
5. Information concerning the influence of the medium used for uterine distention

---

*See references 13, 17, 18, 21, 24, 25, and 31.

Techniques used by different investigators varied from one another by the choice of the distending media, the size and shape of the electrodes, as well as the coagulating power and its length of application (Figs. 11-1 to 11-4). Ten investigators from 5 countries participated in a survey with series ranging from 6 to 298 cases. Of the 778 operations in the survey, 524 patients were tested postoperatively for tubal patency. Following the publication of results[5] that noted failure of the tubes to occlude bilaterally in 33% of the patients and other major complications, the method was not favored. Among the 349 women whose tubes seemed bilaterally occluded on HSG, 11 pregnancies occurred. This finding could indicate recanalization, inadequacy of the tubal patency test, or reopening of the tube by the HSG. The complications included 7 uterine perforations, 8 ectopic pregnancies, 3 intestinal injuries, acute peritonitis in 4 women, and 1 death.[5,15]

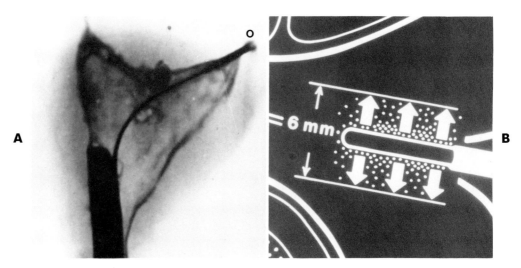

FIG. 11-1 Technique for hysteroscopic electrosurgical sterilization. **A,** Specimen shows probe inserted into uterotubal ostium (*o*). **B,** Schematic representation of depth of insertion, about 6 mm.

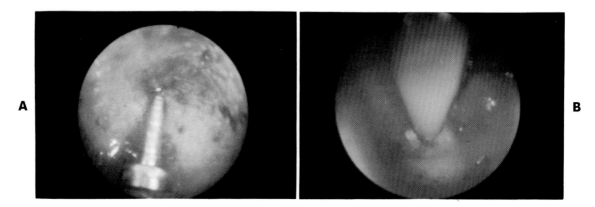

FIG. 11-2 **A,** Probe is ready for insertion into uterotubal ostium. **B,** Electrosurgical coagulation begins. Note whitish periostial area.

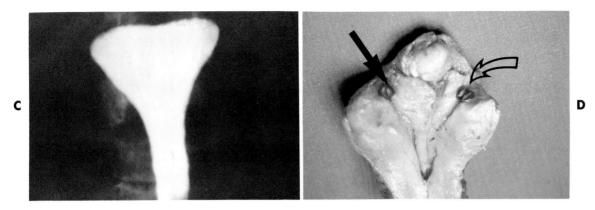

*FIG. Fig. 11-2, cont'd*    **C,** Three months later HSG shows bilateral proximal tubal obstruction but no intramural segment is opacified. **D,** Specimen reveals sites of electrosurgical application (*arrows*).

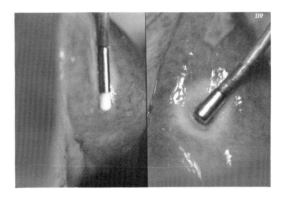

*FIG. 11-3*    Note different reactions of myometrium to two types of probe; one has insulated cap and the other a metal tip.

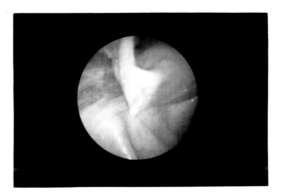

*FIG. 11-4*    Laparoscopic view of hysteroscopic sterilization during electrocoagulation. Note severe thermal effect involving the cornu and isthmus with "near" perforation at uterotubal junction.

Perhaps the most impressive contribution, by Quinones et al.,[25] to the subject of hysteroscopic tubal sterilization appeared in 1976. These authors reported 930 procedures where they used electrosurgical energy. The prerequisites were that the patient had to be in the follicular phase, that an intrauterine pressure of 100 mm Hg be achieved, and that electrocoagulation, with 25 W at the end of the probe for 8 to 10 sec, be precise. The Silastic-tip electrode was inserted 4 to 6 mm into the intramural segment. Vaginitis, cervicitis, myomas, or uterine abnormalities that distorted the cavity were contraindications. The procedure was done using a paracervical block as the local anesthetic. Patients were discharged 20 minutes postoperatively and could resume usual activities the following day. Only one minor complication was reported. Temporary contraception with either an intrauterine device (IUD) or oral contraceptives was advised until a hysterosalpingogram, taken 12 to 14 days postoperatively, confirmed the occlusion. HSGs were performed on 552 patients; 115 women (17.3%) showed unilateral or bilateral patency. These women were resterilized using the same technique and 112 (98%) of them had subsequent bilateral tubal occlusion. No pregnancies occurred in 513 women who had bilateral occlusion and were followed for 1 year. Of the six pregnancies reported by the entire group, three occurred in the interstitial segment. The following factors contributed to failure:

1. Performance of the procedure after day 8 of the cycle
2. Teaching more than one physician at a time and the procedure becoming prolonged
3. The presence of uterine abnormalities
4. Using a ball-tipped electrode
5. Introducing cylindrical-tipped electrodes into the uterotubal ostia for a distance of more than 6 mm
6. Using excessive wattage (>25 W) for long periods of time (more than 10 seconds)

### Sclerosing Agents

Transcervical application or instillation of various chemicals[26] such as gelatin-resorcinol-formaldehyde (GRF),[10] silver nitrate,[33] quinacrine,[25,32] methylcyanoacrylate (MCA),[17,30] phenol-atabrine paste (PAP), and phenol-mucilage[6] and several less promising agents have been used for nonsurgical sterilization. Because quinacrine was recognized as a sclerosing agent, attempts were made to inject it into the fallopian tubes.[25] The usual method involved the injection of 50 to 100 mg. Few complications were reported, but bilateral tubal closure was achieved in only 80% of the patients. The FEMCEPT system requires transcervical introduction of a cannula using a distal balloon. Insufflation positions the tip of the device with lateral openings to instill substances directly into the fallopian tubes without reflux (Fig. 11-5). The device has been designed to deliver 0.6 ml of MCA per instillation. Bilateral tubal closure was achieved in 72% of the tubes after 1 application and in 96% of them with 2 applications 1 month apart.[28]

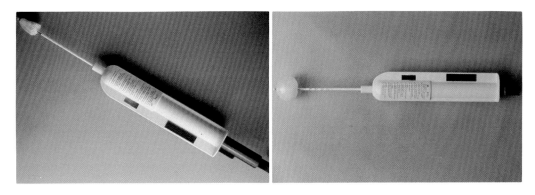

*FIG. 11-5* FEMCEPT device shown before (*a*) and after (*b*) inflation at distal end. (Courtesy A. Goldsmith, MD.)

## Plugs

The use of improved hysteroscopes and accessory instruments has allowed the development and placement of devices and plugs into the intramural segment. The use of silastic formed-in-place plugs involves allowing a catalyzed liquid silicone polymer to flow into the oviduct; the rubber obturator tip positioned at the tubal ostium becomes bonded to the liquid silicone polymer. The resulting flexible structure is larger in diameter at both ends than it is in the isthmus, and it remains in place to effect tubal occlusion. The actual method for the injection of the liquid silicone requires a precise protocol. The solutions must be kept separate until immediately before injection. Once mixed, the injection is accomplished by a screw-driven dispenser.

The sterilization procedure is performed using a local anesthetic. The cervix is dilated and a panoramic hysteroscope is inserted. Hyskon or $CO_2$ can be used as the distention medium. The tubal ostium is identified, the twin catheters are inserted through the operating channel, and the obturator is snugly placed within the tubal ostium. Methylene blue is injected to demonstrate tubal patency and confirm the tight fit. The silicone is mixed with a catalyst and injected after the silicone has been "cured." This curing process takes 4 to 6 minutes. It flows through the inner catheter, the central hole in the obturator, and along the fallopian tube (Fig. 11-6).

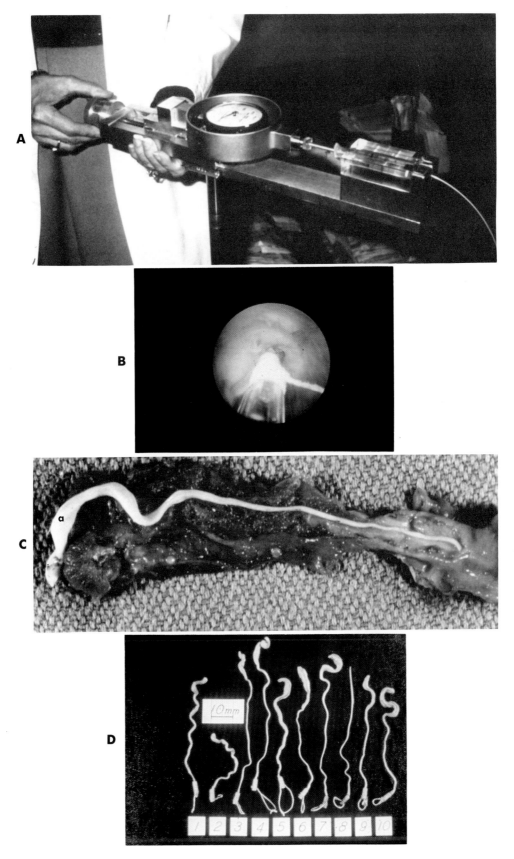

*FIG. 11-6* Technique of hysteroscopic sterilization with formed-in-place silicone plugs. **A,** Silicone has been prepared and administered through specially designed pump. **B,** Plug directed toward uterotubal orifice. **C,** Specimen shows plug in fallopian tube (*a,* ampulla). **D,** Various plugs removed from tubes show different configurations. (Courtesy Theodore P. Reed III, MD.)

Solidification is confirmed in at least 5 minutes. A flatplate x-ray of the pelvis is taken to confirm proper plug formation (Fig. 11-7). The procedure is contraindicated for patients if they have:

- A fixed displaced uterus (retroflexion, retroversion)
- Had a previous term pregnancy less than 6 months ago or an abortion within the last 3 months
- Known tubal abnormalities

Successful sterilizations can be accomplished using the first application for about 80% of the patients.[2,3,7,19,27] The main reasons for failure to achieve sterilization on the first application are tubal spasm, tip separation, and failure to achieve parallel axis (Fig. 11-8). Although the success of HTS using this method has been noteworthy, the need for a follow-up x-ray or HSG to evaluate the continuity of the plug and search for its possible migration is a major disadvantage. Complications other than pregnancy, when improper plugs were used, were few and minor in nature.

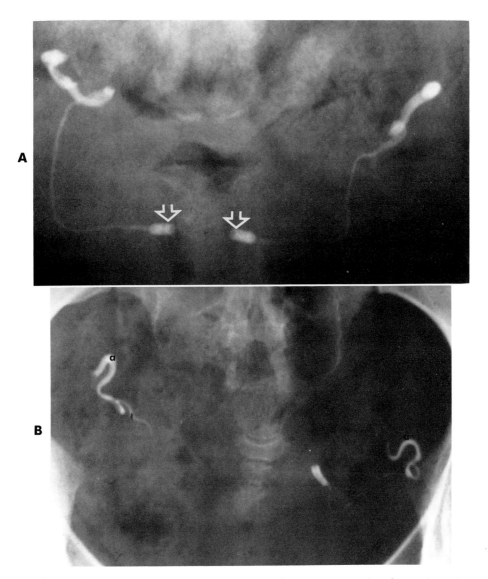

*FIG. 11-7* **A,** Plain x-ray film shows normal, continuous plug formation. *Arrow* indicates uterotubal ostia. **B,** Discontinuous plug is seen (*a,* ampulla).

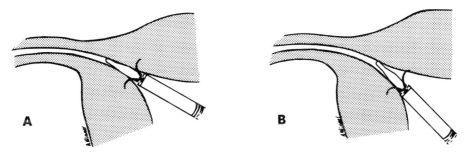

*FIG. 11-8* Parallel axis is essential for good plug placement. **A,** Parallel axis achieved. **B,** Failure to obtain proper alignment.

## Other Mechanical Occlusive Devices

In 1976 Craft[4] reported on the feasibility of the hysteroscopic implantation of ceramic plugs at the uterotubal junction. The porous ceramic plug was supposed to provide a stable support system to allow tissue growth within the porous matrix without causing inflammation or foreign body reactions. The P-block, devised by Brundin,[1] consists of a prefabricated nylon skeleton to which a hydrogelic material has been anchored. The device is placed into the uterotubal ostia under hysteroscopic control through a catheter that also contains a flexible plunger. It is hydrated by body fluids after insertion and retains a good "memory" of the shape during swelling. $CO_2$ was the distending medium used for the hysteroscopic procedure. Other devices[13,23] have been described and used in a few patients but none of the prototypes has been tested in a large enough series for a full evaluation (Fig. 11-9).

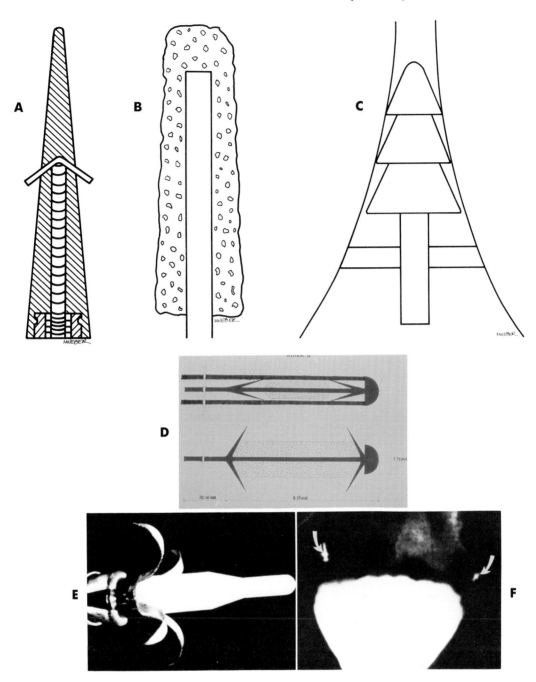

*FIG. 11-9* Tubal plugs. **A,** Brueschke's plug has metallic stiffening core. **B,** Craft's uterotubal ceramic plug. **C,** Sugimoto's silicone rubber intratubal contraceptive device (ITCD). **D,** Brundin's hydrogelic uterotubal plug before hydration (*top*) and after (*bottom*). (Courtesy Jan O. Brundin, MD.) **E,** Hosseinian's plug has metal spines. **F,** Hosseinian plug seen in uterotubal junction on HSG in baboon. (Courtesy Abdol H. Hosseinian, MD.)

Hamou et al.[12] evaluated an intratubal device (ITD) that consisted of a soft strand of nylon 1 mm in diameter. At each end there was a loop with an "elastic memory" (Fig. 11-10). The loop prevented expulsion of the device into either the uterine or peritoneal cavity. Hysteroscopy was performed and the ITD (intratubal device) inserted using a local anesthetic, and $CO_2$ was used to distend the uterine cavity (Fig. 11-11). After 6 months of follow-up for 1471 cycles only 1 intrauterine pregnancy was reported, but 5% of the women could not have the device inserted, and in 15% at least 1 ITD was expelled.[12] Although the technique appears to be safe and relatively easy, significant limitations exist which prevent widespread application. Undoubtedly a major attraction of the nondestructive plug method is the potential for later reversibility.

## SUMMARY

Despite the attractive features of HTS and the painstaking efforts by many investigators in the last decade, the ideal hysteroscopic method is yet to be developed. Mechanical occlusive devices have been an interesting approach but the factors of placement, retention, and complications remain to be evaluated. With all nondestructive plugs and devices, the occurrence of intrauterine and ectopic pregnancy, and the potential for reversibility remain to be evaluated. Electrocoagulation of the tubal cornua was associated with an unacceptably high failure rate and both major and minor complications. The problems of recanalization and extrauterine pregnancies are additional disturbing features.

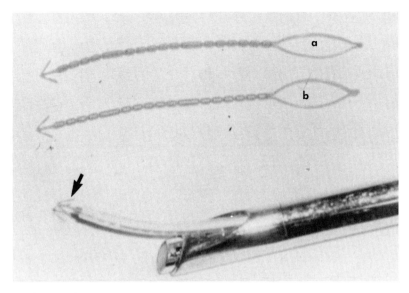

FIG. 11-10  Intratubal device (ITD) consists of loops (*a,b*) with elastic "memory" in nylon strand, 28 to 30 mm long (*upper*). "Spines" (*arrow*) project from end of hysteroscopic sheath.

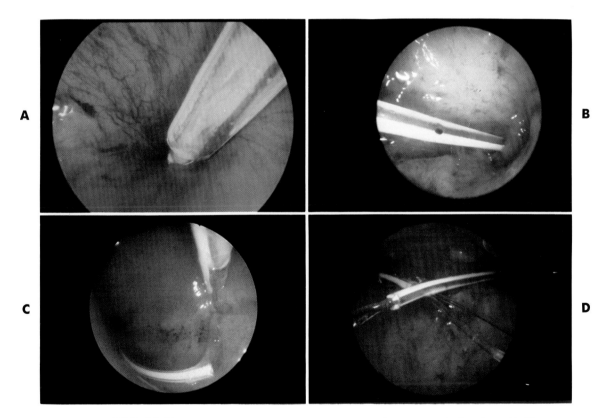

FIG. 11-11  **A,** Cannula containing ITD approaches uterotubal ostium. **B,** Hysteroscopic observation during release of ITD. **C,** ITD has entered uterotubal ostium. **D,** One month later during hysteroscopic examination both loops of ITD can be seen.

*References*

1. Brundin J: Hydrogel tubal blocking device: P-Block. In Zatuchni GI, Shelton JD, Goldsmith A, et al., eds: Female transcervical sterilization, Hagerstown, Md, 1983, Harper & Row.

2. Cooper JM: Hysteroscopic tubal occlusion with formed-in-place silicone plugs. In Sciarra JJ, Zatuchni GI, and Daly M, eds: Gynecology and obstetrics, Hagerstown, Md, 1986, Harper & Row.

3. Corfman PA and Taylor HC: An instrument for transcervical treatment of the oviduct and uterine cornua, Obstet Gynecol 27:880, 1966.

4. Craft I: Uterotubal ceramic plugs. In Sciarra JJ, Droegemueller W, and Speidel JJ, eds: Advances in female sterilization, Hagerstown, Md, 1976, Harper & Row.

5. Darabi KF, Roy K, and Richart RM: Collaborative study on hysteroscopic sterilization procedures: final report. In Sciarra JJ, Zatuchni GI, and Speidel JJ, eds: Risks, benefits and controversies in fertility control, Hagerstown, Md, 1978, Harper & Row.

6. Davis RH, Platt HA, Moonka DK, et al.: Chronic occlusion of the monkey fallopian tube with silicone polymer, Obstet Gynecol 53:527, 1979.

7. De Mayer JFDE: Hysteroscopic sterilization with silicone rubber: A review of 3½ years' experience. In Siegler AM and Lindemann HJ, eds: Hysteroscopy: principles and practice, Philadelphia, 1984, JB Lippincott.

8. Dickinson RL: Simple sterilization of women by cautery stricture at the intrauterine tubal openings, compared with other methods, Surg Obstet Gynecol 23:203, 1916.

9. Droegemueller W, Green BE, Davis JR, et al.: Cryocoagulation of the endometrium at the uterine cornua, Am J Obstet Gynecol 131:1, 1978.

10. Falb RD, Lower BR, Crowley JP, et al.: Transcervical fallopian tube blockage with gelatin-resorcinol-formaldehyde. In Sciarra JJ, Droegemueller W, and Speidel JJ, eds: Advances in female sterilization techniques, Hagerstown, Md, 1976, Harper & Row.

11. Froriep R: Zur Vorbeugung der Notwendigkeit des Kaiserschnitts und der Perforation, Notiz Geb Natur Heilkunde 11:9, 1849.

12. Hamou J, Gasparri F, Cittadini E, et al.: Hysteroscopic placement of nylon intratubal devices for potentially reversible sterilization. In Siegler AM and Ansari AH, eds: The fallopian tube: basic studies and clinical considerations, New York, 1986, Futura.

13. Hosseinian AH: Hysteroscopic sterilization. In Siegler AM and Ansari AH, eds: The fallopian tube: basic studies and clinical considerations, New York, 1986, Futura.

14. Hyams MN: Sterilization of the female by coagulation of the uterine cornu, Am J Obstet Gynecol 28:96, 1934.

15. Israngkun CH and Phoasavsadi S: Hysteroscopy sterilization complications in 269 cases. In Sciarra JJ, Droegemueller W, and Speidel JJ, eds: Advances in female sterilization techniques, Hagerstown, Md, 1976, Harper & Row.

16. Kocks J: Eine neue Methode der Sterilisation der Frauen, Zentralb Gynäkol 2:617, 1878.

17. Lindemann HJ and Mohr J: Tubensterilisation per Hysteroskop, Sexualmedizin 3:1222, 1974.

18. Lindemann HJ, Gallinat A, Lueken RP, et al.: Atlas der Hysteroskopie, Stuttgart, 1980, Gustav Fischer.

19. Loffer FD: Hysteroscopic sterilization with the use of formed-in-place silicone plugs, Am J Obstet Gynecol 149:261, 1984.

20. von Mickulicz-Radecki F and Freund A: Ein neues Hysteroskop und seine praktische Anwendung in der Gynäkologie, Geburtsh Gynäkol 92:13, 1927.

21. Neuwirth RS, Richart RM, Israngkun CH, et al.: Hysteroscopic sterilization. In Sciarra JJ, Butler JC, and Speidel JJ, eds: Hysteroscopic sterilization, New York, 1974, Intercontinental Medical Book Corp.

22. Norment WB, Sikes CH, Berry FX, and Bird I: Hysteroscopy, Surg Clin North Am 37:1377, 1957.

23. Popp LW, Schulz S, and Lindemann HJ: Intratubal devices in rats: An experimental model. In Siegler AM and Lindemann HJ, eds: Hysteroscopy: principles and practice, Philadelphia, 1984, JB Lippincott.

24. Quinones RG, Aznar RR, and Duran HA: Tubal electrocauterization under hysteroscopic control, Contraception 7:195, 1973.
25. Quinones RG, Alvarado DA, and Ley E: Hysteroscopic sterilization, Int J Gynaecol Obstet 14:27, 1976.
26. Rakshit B: The scope of liquid plastics and other chemicals for blocking the fallopian tubes. In Richart RM and Prager DJ, eds: Human sterilization, Springfield, IL, 1972, Charles C Thomas.
27. Reed TP and Erb RA: Hysteroscopic occlusion with silicone rubber, Obstet Gynecol 61:388, 1983.
28. Richart RM, Neuwirth RS, Nilsen PA, et al.: The effectiveness of FEM-CEPT method and preliminary experience with radio-opaque MCA to enhance clinical acceptability. In Zatuchni GI, Shelton JD, Goldsmith A, et al., eds: Female transcervical sterilization, Hagerstown, Md, 1983, Harper & Row.
29. Schroeder C: Über den Aufbau und die Leistungen der Hysteroskopie, Arch Gynäkol 156:407, 1934.
30. Stevenson TC and Taylor DS: The effect of methyl cyanoacrylate tissue adhesive on the human fallopian tube and endometrium, J Obstet Gynaecol Br Emp 79:1028, 1972.
31. Sugimoto O: Diagnostic and therapeutic hysteroscopy, Tokyo, 1978, Igaku-Shoin.
32. Zipper J, Mendel M, Pastene L, et al.: Intrauterine instillation of chemical cytotoxic agents for tubal sterilization and treatment of functional metrorrhagias, Int J Fertil 14:280, 1969.
33. Zipper JA, Stachetti E, and Mendel M: Human fertility control by transvaginal application of quinacrine on the fallopian tube, Fertil Steril 21:581, 1970.

# 12 *Chorionic Villi Sampling*

Amniocentesis is a low-risk, remarkably accurate procedure used to ascertain a prenatal genetic diagnosis. Some disadvantages are the following:

1. The limited time during gestation that the procedure can be safely performed
2. The subsequent waiting period
3. The few elective terminations of pregnancy performed mostly between 18 to 22 weeks' of gestation
4. The advent of fetal movement and the incipient fetal-maternal bonding
5. The risks inherent in late second trimester abortion

The advantage of taking chorionic villi samples (CVS) rather than doing an amniocentesis to diagnose genetic disorders is that the specimens can be processed during the first trimester of pregnancy. It is possible to obtain pure cultures of rapidly growing fetal cells for cytogenetic analysis by transcervical biopsy or aspiration techniques. Fetal sex determination (preferably for sex-linked diseases only) can be accomplished in 3 to 4 days, and chromosomal analysis can be determined within 2 weeks of the biopsy. Molecular genetic techniques, utilizing restriction endonucleases, have allowed successful prenatal diagnosis of sickle cell anemia and thalassemia. The amount of DNA procured from these specimens has been ample for such determinations.[22]

## ANATOMY OF THE CHORION AND DECIDUA

The chorion, the outermost fetal membrane, is a multilayered structure that consists of a somatic mesoderm and a trophoblast. It is the most accessible fetal tissue, obvious in the first trimester when villi are distributed over the entire chorionic membrane (Fig. 12-1). Fetal blood vessels supply the villi (Fig. 12-2). The chorion frondosum contain villi that touch the decidua basalis and form the future placenta.

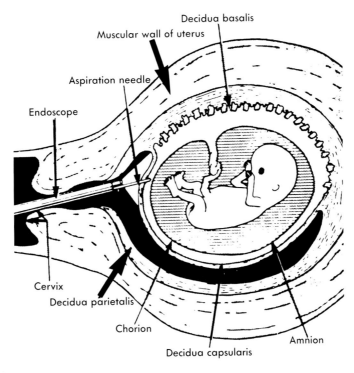

*FIG. 12-1* Schematic representation shows relationship of fetal membranes, villi, and decidual layers. (From Rodeck CH and Morsman JM: Br Med Bull 39:338, 1983.)

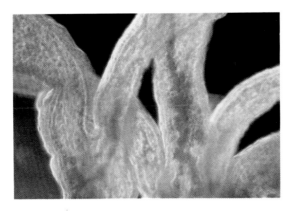

*FIG. 12-2* During hysteroscopic examination, fetal vessels are clearly seen in chorionic villi.

The decidua capsularis is the superficial decidual layer that covers the entire fetal sac, but it gradually fuses with the decidua parietalis opposite it and obliterates the endometrial cavity in the third or fourth month as the gestational sac grows (Fig. 12-3). The attached villi atrophy when their circulation becomes impaired. The extraplacental chorion eventually is denuded of villi and becomes the chorion laeve.

With CVS, the trophoblastic fetal tissue is removed from the chorionic frondosum between the seventh and twelfth week of gestation. Until recently most chorionic villi were aspirated by a catheter inserted into the area of the chorionic frondosum using ultrasonic guidance.

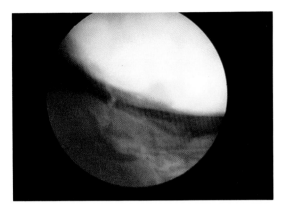

*FIG. 12-3* In a 12-week gestation, amniotic sac approaches decidua parietalis, almost obliterating cavity.

## INDICATIONS

The need for a prenatal diagnosis is indicated when the physician thinks the developing embryo has an increased risk of a biochemical or chromosomal defect. Fetal genetic aberrations such as Down syndrome (trisomy 21), hemoglobinopathies (sickle cell disease), metabolic errors (Tay-Sachs disease), and aneuploidy can be discovered by amniocentesis or CVS. Neural tube defects, such as spina bifida, should be suspected when there is a change in the level of $\alpha$-fetoprotein in the amniotic fluid, but these defects are not evident in villi or amniotic cells.

Chromosomal analysis of the embryo should be done under the following circumstances:[13]

1. Advanced maternal age; mother will be more than 35 years old at the time of delivery
2. The patient, the partner, or a close relative delivered a child with chromosomal problems such as Down syndrome
3. Either parent is a known carrier of a chromosomal disorder (mosaicism or translocation)
4. Mother is a known or suspected carrier of a sex-linked disease (hemophilia or Duchenne muscular dystrophy)
5. One or both parents are carriers of a recessive gene (Tay-Sachs)

Transcervical sampling is possible either by removal of tissue by aspiration through a fine needle or with biopsy forceps under echographic[3,9] or endoscopic control.[4-6] Ultrasound guided techniques include insertion of either an aspiration polyethylene catheter[23] that has an echogenic metal strip in its wall, or a biopsy forceps inserted into the cervical canal. Ultrasonic techniques have made CVS safer, simpler, and more accurate because of new, high-resolution equipment (Fig. 12-4).

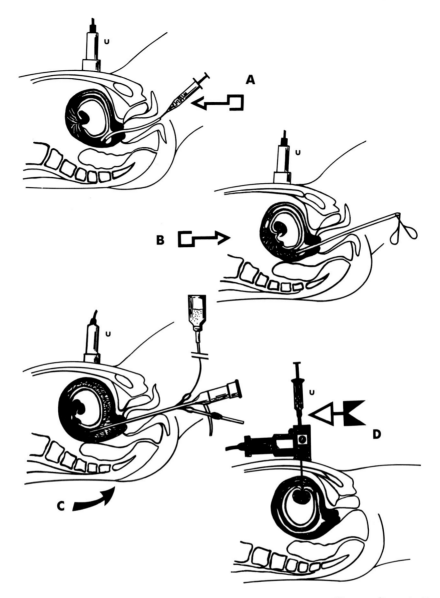

***FIG. 12-4*** Ultrasound (*u*) guided techniques for chorionic villi sampling. **A,** Transcervical needle aspiration. **B,** Transcervical biopsy forceps. **C,** Hysteroscopic guided biopsy forceps. **D,** Transabdominal needle aspiration.

## HYSTEROSCOPICALLY GUIDED CVS

Since 1970, when clinical hysteroscopic methods and concepts were first used, various devices and technical modifications have been developed to obtain chorionic villi. A medium, either gas or liquid, was required to distend the uterine cavity and separate the lens of the hysteroscope from the tissue.[19] However, in many instances, the decidua capsularis was pushed against the chorionic tissue, and the distending media and villi could only be seen after a small piece of decidua had been removed.

Endoscopic CVS was described initially by Hahnemann and Mohr[8] and Hahnemann[7] for patients scheduled for immediate or delayed (8 days) termination of pregnancy. In the karyotypes obtained from about one third of the procedures the analysis of biopsy specimen cultures showed the same chromosomal constitution as fetuses after subsequent abortion. Complications occurred as the result of puncture and laceration of the amniotic sac; intrauterine bleeding obscured the gynecologist's vision in several instances. As the technique has improved it has become possible to avoid contamination of trophoblastic material with the maternal tissues, to select properly vascularized villi, and to locate areas of the chorion that have abundant surface villi.

Rodeck and Morsman[18] assessed 6 biopsy techniques done for 45 patients in their first trimester of pregnancy, including blind aspiration biopsy using several types of cannulas (Fig. 12-5), biopsy forceps used with contact hysteroscopy, biopsy forceps used under direct vision with and without ultrasound control, and aspiration biopsy used under direct vision with and without ultrasound control. They discovered the combination of ultrasound, a transcervical endoscope, and an aspiration needle was the most successful method, and no maternal or fetal complications were noted.

Kullander and Sandhal[12] devised a 5 mm endocerviscope through which a biopsy forceps could be inserted. Gustavii[6] used a fetoscope, 1.7 mm in diameter, a biopsy forceps, and saline solution to distend the uterine cavity. CVS was done 1 to 2 cm from the edge of the placenta. Nordenskjold and Gustavii[17] used a 4.7 mm OD sheathed endoscope with 2 attachments, 1 for the instillation of NS at body temperature and the other for a biopsy forceps. The extraembryonic sac was distended with NS and the biopsy forceps were used to remove a piece of decidua near the edge of the placenta. To avoid contamination from maternal tissue adhering to the jaws of the first biopsy forceps it was replaced with another one, and specimens were taken from the edge of the placenta. Fetal heart activity was monitored before, during, and after the procedure. The technique was used for 21 patients and 19 pregnancies went to term. One patient had a miscarriage 3 weeks after the procedure. The specimens obtained were sufficient for karyotyping (fetal sex determination for suspected sex-linked disorders) by direct preparation in 3 of 17 cases. The remaining specimens were allowed to culture for 2 to 3 weeks. The material taken was insufficient for measuring enzymes.

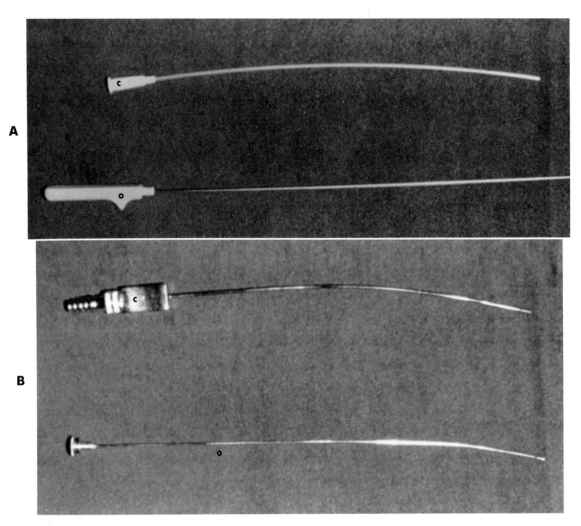

*FIG. 12-5* Two aspiration cannulas used with ultrasonic guidance for CVS. **A,** Portex catheter (*c*) has 1.5 mm OD and is 21 cm in length, is plastic with removable stainless steel obturator (*o*). **B,** Down's cannula is made of 16 gauge silver tubing and measures 23 cm in length. It also has obturator (*o*).

Ghirardini et al.[4] named their endoscope a chorionoscope (Fig. 12-6). The chamber tip could collect a 30 mg specimen of villi. Ultrasound was performed preoperatively to ascertain the gestational age and localize the placenta.[7] The collecting chamber was kept closed until the instrument passed the internal os. As it moved toward the placental site a small amount of NS (5 ml) was instilled and, once the villi were seen they were aspirated into the collecting chamber with the same syringe used for fluid injection.[2] With this device, the visibility was good enough to allow the physicians to distinguish between villi of the chorion frondosum and atrophic villi of the chorion laeve. Because of the large diameter of the chorionoscope (4 mm), placental abruption was a theoretic possibility. Chorionoscopy was attempted on 70 patients and quality villi were obtained in 63 instances. After CVS 7 (10%) of the patients aborted. The tenth week of gestation is considered as the ideal time to perform the procedure. Contraindications to chorionoscopy were bleeding in pregnancy, vaginal infection, myoma, IUD in situ, and a retroverted uterus with a posterior placenta.

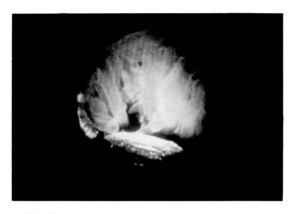

*FIG. 12-6* Villi can be seen through Ghirardini chorionoscope and selected for CVS.

Another approach for CVS is the window hysteroscopic technique.[16] An ultrasound examination was done preoperatively to obtain precise information about the duration of gestation and location of the placenta. The bladder was emptied and the hysteroscope inserted into the endocervical canal under visual control (Fig. 12-7). Echographic control should not be used because the $CO_2$ flow into the uterine cavity would distort the image. An insufflator was used to distend the uterine cavity with $CO_2$ at a flowrate of 30 ml/min to maintain intrauterine pressure below 10 mm Hg. It was not necessary to dilate the cervical canal or to use any anesthesia. When the isthmus was reached, 20 to 30 seconds elapsed to allow the uterine cavity to distend completely.

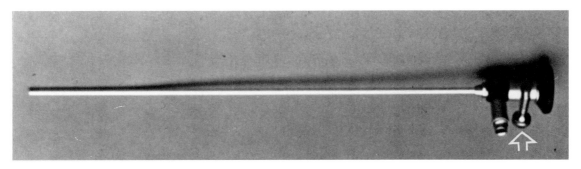

*FIG. 12-7* Hysteroscope is 3 mm in diameter and 35 cm in length, has focusing knob (*arrow*) near the ocular lens, and is inserted into 5 mm sheath.

The greenish gestational sac became clearly visible as it protruded into the uterine cavity (Fig. 12-8). When the placental insertion and the reflection of the decidua capsularis onto the uterine wall were located, a 2 cm "window" was opened. Trauma to superficial decidual vessels must be avoided to prevent the formation of a postoperative decidual hematoma. The opening was cut and then a forceps inserted for a depth of 0.5 to 1 cm to take a tissue specimen.

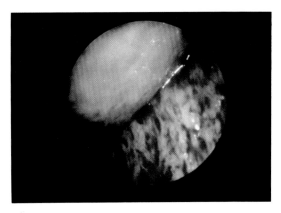

*FIG. 12-8* Greenish gestational sac of 10 weeks' gestation is juxtaposed to decidua parietalis.

The lens remained outside the gestational sac and only a minimal amount of $CO_2$ entered the uterine cavity (Fig. 12-9). As the biopsy forceps was removed, the endoscopist made a visual inspection of the quantity and quality of the sample after which it was promptly examined microscopically to verify adequacy (Fig. 12-10).

Mencaglia et al.[16] performed this operation on 112 patients who had requested termination of pregnancy. (The reported series did not include 30 patients who had undergone the technique to enable the physicians to perfect the method). In 110 instances it was possible to insert the hysteroscope into the uterine cavity without any local or general anesthesia, or dilating of the cervical canal; in 2 patients, the examination was not possible because of cervical stenosis. The technique was successful for 110 patients because the material removed was chorionic villi, uncontaminated by decidual tissue. The patients were sent home the same day and were requested to return in 1 week for another ultrasound examination prior to termination of pregnancy. During the first postoperative week two miscarriages occurred. Ultrasound, in the remaining 108 patients, revealed a normal gestational sac with fetal cardiac activity and no retroplacental hematomas. Of these women 4 reported feeling some abdominal pain for 4 to 6 hours after sampling, and 39 patients suffered from slight vaginal bleeding for a few days.

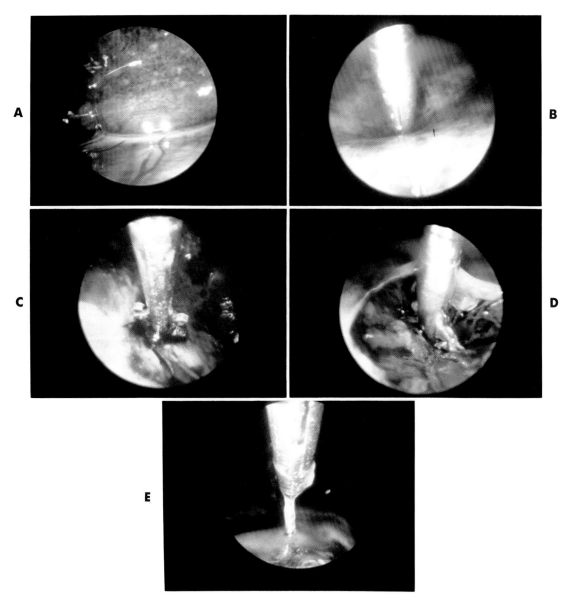

FIG. 12-9 Window technique for CVS. A, Gestational sac is lying on decidua parietalis. B, Part of gestational sac is being pushed off decidua parietalis. C, Biopsy forceps inserted, jaws are opened to expose chorionic villi. D, Through decidual window chorionic villi become visible. E, CVS is taken in forceps.

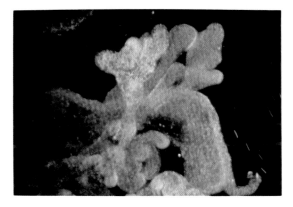

FIG. 12-10 Chorionic villi observed at ×40 magnification.

## ULTRASONIC GUIDED CVS

Thus far only a small percentage of CVS procedures have been performed by endoscopic techniques with continuing pregnancies. Pregnancy had been considered a relative contraindication to hysteroscopy. Holzegreve and Miney[9] used hysteroscopy before and after CVS to evaluate the degree of trauma caused by various techniques. More bleeding seemed to result from samples taken under endoscopic control than from catheter aspiration procedures. Based on experience they decided to use the catheter technique guided sonographically to reach the chorion frondosum. After withdrawal of the obturator, a 20 ml syringe was attached to the catheter and suction applied. In all instances, the amount of villi was sufficient for chromosomal analysis after the villi were cultured. The banding quality of chromosomes following culture was as good as after amniotic fluid cultures.

Ultrasonic guided CVS using transcervical aspiration has been the most widely used method and provides success in 98% of the cases,[2,11] but it has certain limitations.

1. It cannot locate precisely the decidua capsularis or the best insertion site for the aspiration cannula to avoid superficial vessels (Fig. 12-11).
2. If the sampling catheter ruptures the decidua, the biopsy specimen can become contaminated with deciduous maternal tissue and confuse the cytogenetic findings.
3. The pressure needed by the catheter to overcome resistance of the decidual wall can traumatize the amniotic sac causing a spontaneous abortion.

With transabdominal CVS, the sampling is not performed through the cervix, possible vaginal contamination is avoided, and it is easy to move the probe in the abdomen. Maxwell et al.[15] and Smidt-Jensen et al.[20] stated they were able to remove 30 mg of villous material by the transabdominal route. Bovicelli et al.[1] indicated it was possible to perform a cytogenetic analysis in only 52% of chorionic specimens obtained in this manner, but this figure reached 82% when the sample was obtained transcervically. MacKenzie et al.[14] were able to withdraw 10 mg of villi in only 26% of the patients with transabdominal CVS, but in 70% using the transcervical route. Jackson[10] collected data from 92 centers and concluded that only 1% to 5% of all CVSs had been obtained by the abdominal route. The method is readily accepted by the patients, it has a high success rate, and the innovation of the negative pressure pumps has made it possible to obtain a sufficient quantity of tissue for genetic and enzymatic analysis. Use of negative pressure pumps may negate the inadequate samples obtained transabdominally.

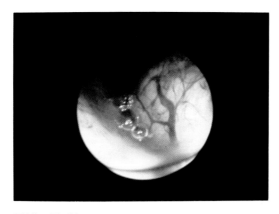

*FIG. 12-11*  Superficial vessels in gestational sac, to be avoided during CVS.

## RISKS OF CHORIONIC VILLI SAMPLING

The safety of this relatively new procedure has been well established from the report in the International Registry. Over 7000 chorionic villi samplings have been performed in 72 centers, and there were 56 (0.8%) failed samples, 566 (8.0%) therapeutic abortions, and 6583 continuing pregnancies.[10] The rate of fetal loss was 3.8% and 2321 patients delivered. If one adds the risk of amniocentesis to the percentage of pregnancies that would spontaneously abort by the sixteenth week, the rate of fetal loss associated with CVS is under 4%. Few postoperative infections have been reported, and incorrect karyotyping was rare, but with cultured cell preparations this error is eliminated.

Several studies have been done to compare the risks from CVS with those from amniocentesis. Smidt-Jensen et al.[20] noted 10 fetal losses from 208 patients who had transabdominal CVS compared to 2 from 195 cases of amniocentesis; moreover CVS failed in 6 cases and amniocentesis in 2. They compared the incidence of pregnancy wastage from transabdominal CVS, transcervical CVS, and amniocentesis (Table 12-1).

CVS has minimal risks and is successful most of the time for solving the prenatal problem. Failed cell cultures, unanalyzable metaphases because of condensed chromosomes, and difficult banding are problems being overcome with advances in technology. One could argue that almost all trisomies (over 97%) will be aborted spontaneously and second trimester amniocentesis for prenatal diagnosis will reveal those few trisomies that escape the body's natural surveillance and defense system. Those first trimester abnormal embryos already destined to spontaneously abort could include those normal embryos whose loss or damage was induced by the CVS diagnostic procedure.

*Table 12-1* Comparison of Transabdominal CVS, Transcervical CVS, and Amniocentesis[21]

|  | Transabdominal CVS | Transcervical CVS | Amniocentesis |
|---|---|---|---|
| Randomized | 272 | 278 | 296 |
| Withdrew before procedure | 2 | 6 | 13 |
| Fetal loss before procedure | 2 | 3 | 9 |
|  | 268 | 269 | 274 |
| Randomized procedure performed | 264 | 235 | 274 |
| Repeated/other procedure | 4 | 34 | 0 |
| Fetal loss after procedure | 9 | 15 | 2 |
| Elective abortion | 10 | 4 | 4 |

From Smidt-Jensen S, Philip J: Transabdominal CVS vs transcervical CVS amniocentesis. Randomized study: International Conference on Chorionic Villus Sampling and Early Prenatal Diagnosis, Athens, Greece, May 28-29, 1988.

## SUMMARY

There are many potential applications for chorionic biopsy as a prenatal diagnostic procedure. Currently chromosomal analysis is the major application. First trimester chorionic biopsy has the potential to replace the diagnostic genetic amniocentesis. The advantage of being able to make prenatal diagnoses of chromosomal abnormalities in the first trimester instead of the second trimester (when amniocentesis is used) is obvious. The information gained about the early chorion through direct examination by hysteroscopy has contributed to our knowledge about trophoblastic tissue. The optimal sampling techniques are yet to evolve, and the best technical method for chromosomal analyses are being established. This technique has been used in DNA analysis to determine the presence of sickle cell disease and thalassemia.

Chorionic villi sampling is reliable, the fetal loss rate is about 4%, and failed samples occur in only 3%. Potential problems include contamination of trophoblastic material with maternal tissue and blood, damage to the amniotic membrane, bleeding, and infection.

CVS can be performed early in pregnancy by combining ultrasonic guidance with direct vision endoscopic biopsy. The hysteroscopic method requires the physician to have extensive experience in avoiding sequelae and obtaining adequate samples for analysis. The hysteroscopic technique remains experimental. Although the diagnostic possibilities are recognized, its clinical applicability has yet to be ascertained. The amount of placental tissue exceeds the volume of the fetus in the first 8 to 10 weeks, making the procedure practical.

*References*

1. Bovicelli L, Rizzo N, Montacuti V, et al.: Transabdominal versus transcervical routes for chorionic villus sampling (letter), Lancet 2:290, 1986.
2. Brambati B, Oldrini A, Ferrazzi E, et al.: Chorionic villi sampling: general methodological and clinical approach. In Fraccaro M, Simoni G, and Brambati B, eds: First trimester fetal diagnosis, Berlin, 1985, Springer-Verlag.
3. Dumez Y, Goossens M, Booue J, et al.: Chorionic villi sampling using rigid forceps under ultrasound control. In Fraccaro M, Simoni G, and Brambati B, eds: First trimester fetal diagnosis, Berlin, 1985, Springer-Verlag.
4. Ghirardini G, Gualerzi C, Fochi L, et al.: Chorionoscopy and chorionic villi, Acta Eur Fertil 17:495, 1986.
5. Gustavii B: First trimester chromosomal analysis of chorionic villi obtained by direct vision technique, Lancet 2:507, 1983.
6. Gustavii B: Direct vision technique for chorionic villi sampling in diagnostic cases. In Fraccaro M, Simoni G, and Brambati B, eds: First trimester fetal diagnosis, Berlin, 1985, Springer-Verlag.
7. Hahnemann H: Early prenatal diagnosis: A study of biopsy techniques and cell culturing from extraembryonic membranes, Clin Genet 6:294, 1974.
8. Hahnemann H and Mohr J: Antenatal foetal diagnosis in genetic disease, Bull Eur Soc Hum Genet 3:47, 1969.
9. Holzegreve N, Miney P, Stening C, et al.: Experience with different techniques of chorionic villi sampling for first trimester diagnosis, Acta Eur Fertil 17:485, 1986.
10. Jackson L: Chorionic villus sampling. CVS latest news: fetal loss, Philadelphia, 1985, Thomas Jefferson University Medical College.
11. Kazy Z, Rozoovsky IS, and Bakharev VA: Chorion biopsy in early pregnancy: a method of early diagnosis of inherited disorders, Prenat Diagn 2:29, 1982.
12. Kullander S and Sandhal B: Fetal chromosome analysis after transcervical placental biopsies during early pregnancies, Acta Obstet Gynecol Scand 52:355, 1973.
13. Ludomirsky A and Librizzi R: Chorionic villi sampling, a prenatal diagnosis, Postgrad Obstet Gynecol 6:1, 1986.
14. MacKenzie A, Holmes DS, and Newton JR: A study comparing transcervical with transabdominal chorionic villus sampling (CVS), Br J Obstet Gynaecol 95:75, 1988.
15. Maxwell D, Lilford R, Czepulkowski B, et al.: Transabdominal chorionic villus sampling, Lancet 2:123, 1986.
16. Mencaglia L, Ricci G, Perino A, et al.: Hysteroscopic chorionic villi sampling: a new approach, Acta Eur Fertil 17:491, 1986.
17. Nordenskjold F and Gustavii B: Direct vision chorionic villi biopsy for prenatal diagnosis in the first trimester, J Reprod Med 29:572, 1984.
18. Rodeck CH and Morsman JM: First-trimester chorion biopsy, Br Med Bull 39:338, 1983.
19. Scarselli G, Mencaglia L, and Hamou J: Atlante di microcolpoisteroscopia, Palermo, 1982, COFESE.
20. Smidt-Jensen S, Hahnemann N, Harir J, et al.: Transabdominal chorionic villus sampling for first trimester fetal diagnosis. First 26 pregnancies followed to term, Prenat Diagn 6:125, 1986.
21. Smidt-Jensen S, Philip J: Transabdominal CVS vs transcervical CVS amniocentesis. Randomized study: International Conference on Chorionic Villus Sampling and Early Prenatal Diagnosis, Athens, Greece, May 28-29, 1988.
22. Upadaya M, Archer LM, Harper PS, et al.: DNA and enzyme studies on chorionic villi for use in antenatal diagnosis, Clin Chem Acta 140:239, 1984.
23. Ward RHT, Modell B, Petrou M, et al.: Chorionic villi sampling in a high-risk population using the Portex cannula. In Fraccaro M, Simoni G, and Brambati B, eds: First trimester fetal diagnosis, Berlin, 1985, Springer-Verlag.

# 13 *Documentation*

An easy, quick, and inexpensive method for recording findings from the hysteroscopic examination is a written report of the procedure that is immediately available for future reference and review. This report can be included in the patient's chart. A schematic representation, photographs, and video recordings can be included to aid the surgeon in evaluating the effectiveness of treatment.

The written report and the drawing should be done at the conclusion of each procedure and not at the end of the physician's schedule for the day. The most accurate record is available when the operative procedure is still fresh in the surgeon's mind. Such a document should include the patient's history and results of the physical and pelvic examination. Any pertinent test results such as the hysterosalpingogram should be noted. Other essentials are: the reasons for the hysteroscopic procedure, the type of anesthesia used, whether cervical dilatation was necessary, and the date of the patient's last menses. The written account of the hysteroscopic procedure should include the type and quantity of the distending medium, the method of instillation, and the characteristics of the uterine cavity describing in a systematic manner the anterior, posterior, and lateral walls of the endometrium, the cornua, the uterotubal ostia, and the endocervical canal (Fig. 13-1). All abnormal findings should be documented in detail.

**Hysteroscopic Examination**

NAME _____ AGE _____ DATE _____ LMP _____

      Parity _____

MENSES: Regular _____ Irregular _____     UTERUS: Anterior _____
                                                          Posterior _____
                                                          Size: Normal _____
                                                                Enlarged _____

PREVIOUS PELVIC OPERATIONS:
HSG: Date _____ Result _____

INDICATION: _____

---

ANESTHESIA: No _____ Yes _____ Type _____     Medium _____

Cervical dilatation: No _____ Yes _____

FUNDUS: Normal _____ Abnormality _____

Cornu
  Left _____ Right _____
Ostium
  Left _____ Right _____
Lateral wall
  Left _____ Right _____

ANTERIOR WALL _____     POSTERIOR WALL _____

ENDOCERVICAL CANAL _____

---

DIAGNOSIS: Normal cavity
           Abnormality

COMPLICATIONS:

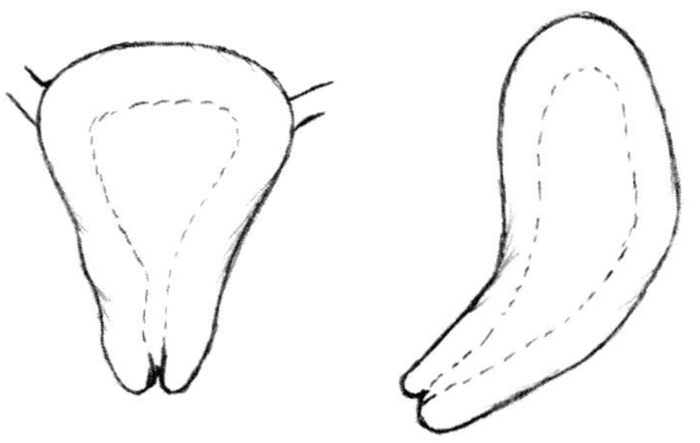

FIG. *13-1* Suggested form for recording data of hysteroscopic findings.

## STILL PHOTOGRAPHY

Single lens reflex (SLR) cameras can be adapted for endoscopic photography. The operator must be able to attach the camera securely to the eyepiece of the hysteroscope, hold both pieces of equipment steady, and view clearly the area of interest. Customized, specially designed cameras are also available for taking 35 mm endoscopic photographs. The camera should be equipped with an automatic exposure meter, motor driven, and capable of having the date recorded on the film (Fig. 13-2). The ground glass focusing screen, a feature of most SLR cameras, should be replaced with a clear glass screen for better viewing.

The focal length of the lens determines the amount the film frame can be filled with an object and the brightness of the image. The longer the lens the darker the image. A zoom lens with focal lengths varying from 70 mm to 140 mm is the most versatile (Fig. 13-3). In all instances, a circular picture is produced.

Most endoscopic photography requires color film that is balanced for electronic flash, designated as daylight film, which emphasizes the blue light spectrum, with temperatures that are in the 5,000° to 6,000° range. For 35 mm cameras with flash units, 200 to 400 ASA, daylight slide film is preferable. Although prints can be made from slides, there is loss of detail, but they can be included with the patient's permanent record. Unexposed film can be preserved in a refrigerator and should be loaded in subdued light.

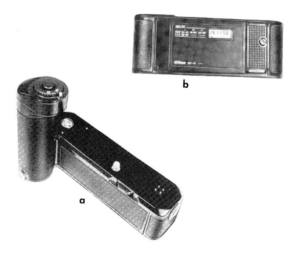

*FIG. 13-2* Motor-driven winder (*a*) is used for automatic transport of film for single or rapid sequential photographs. Data back (*b*) can record information on the film.

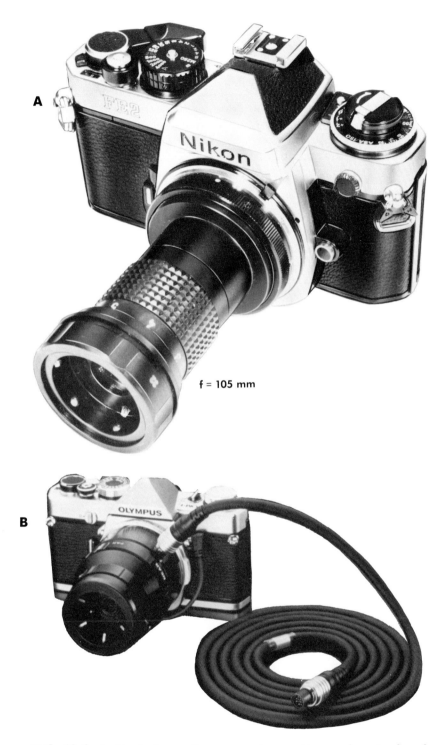

f = 105 mm

*FIG. 13-3* **A,** Single-lens reflex camera has continuous focusing lens for still photography. **B,** Camera is equipped with OM adapter, SM-ER 2 Olympus focusing lens, and cable for flash photography.

## Light Sources

The proximal flash can give accurate exposures from $\frac{1}{100}$ to $\frac{1}{300}$/second and recycle in 2 seconds (Fig. 13-4). The settings on each light source and on the camera must be adjusted carefully in accordance with the instruction manual. Fiberoptic cables transmit the light from the source to the endoscope and operative field. The length of the cable, the number of interface junctions in the course of the fiberoptic bundle, the size of the endoscope, and the cable condition influence the amount of light available for photographic exposure. The use of liquid cables is no longer essential to increase light transmission. They were found to be deficient in the red end of the spectrum and are heavier and more expensive than the newer fiber lightguides.

One camera that is available has the electronic flash generator attached to a fiberoptic cable which is connected to a flashcube. The flashcube is encased in plastic housing that provides 1 outlet and a connection for the examining light. This cube sits securely on the endoscope lightpost and camera synchronization is supplied by a cable (Fig. 13-5).

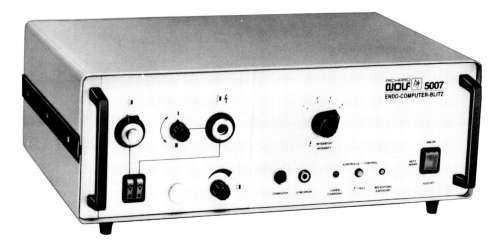

*FIG. 13-4* Generator automatically controls duration of flash and uses optical and acoustical signals.

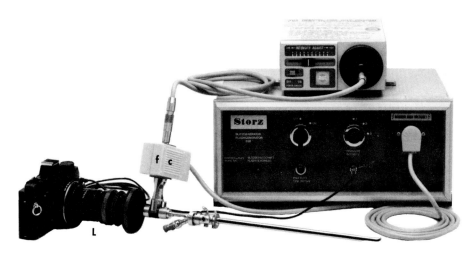

*FIG. 13-5* Camera and focusing lens (*l*) attached to hysteroscope. Flashcube (*fc*) is inserted between fiberoptic light cable and lightpost of hysteroscope.

**PHOTOGRAPHER'S CHECKLIST**

1. Note the shutter speed and check the motor drive. Set the ASA to correspond with the film speed and determine the number of unexposed films that are available.
2. Clean the lens of the camera and the endoscope ocular lens; be certain they are compatible. Set lens focus to infinity.
3. Turn the light source on, test the electronic flash generator, and attach the lightcables to their appropriate site on the scope.
4. Establish a clear hysteroscopic view, attach the camera, check through the viewfinder, and take multiple exposures, preferably with a motor driven/data-back attachment.

   Planning is important. Take several photographs because film is inexpensive and specific selected abnormalities might not be seen again.

**STERILIZATION/DISINFECTION**

Some video cameras and cables can be disinfected by soaking them in a glutaraldehyde (Cidex) solution, but the photographic camera cannot be disinfected this way. Changing gloves can be an alternative whenever before and after therapeutic procedures have to be photographed.

**VIDEO**

Videohysteroscopy is a valuable method for monitoring procedures that involve the Nd:YAG laser because retinal damage from backscattering is avoided, and the gynecologist does not need to use special protective goggles. Furthermore the observation of systematic laser ablation of the endometrium, with adequate observation and comfort for the operator, is facilitated. Although the field of view is reduced and precision may be decreased, this can be overcome with experience. Use of a beam-splitter enables direct viewing through the endoscope, and occasional observation is possible on the video screen (Fig. 13-6). Even when using a beam splitter, protective goggles must be worn if the Nd:YAG laser is used.

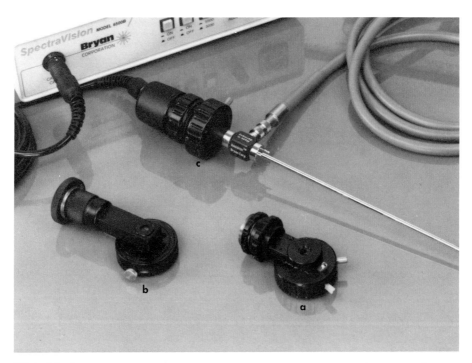

*FIG. 13-6* Beam-splitters simultaneously allow a direct view by gynecologist and video monitoring. **A,** 50-50 beam-splitter. **B,** 30-70 beam-splitter. **C,** Coupling device interfaces between ocular lens of endoscope and video camera.

## Cameras

A good video camera should be small, easy to handle, and lightweight. The sensor should be capable of delivering over 300 lines of resolution and should provide crisp, natural-color renditions even in low light, and orientation should be recognizable by touch. The camera should be sterilized with ethylene oxide or completely disinfected by immersing it in an appropriate solution. Filmless photography is possible using a microcomputer chip; the charged coupled device (CCD) sensor. This small, solid-state unit contains thousands of light sensitive elements called pixels, and the images are converted to video signals which are transmitted to the tape. Some of the cameras weigh only 60 g and are only 2.4 cm in diameter. Fine-adjustment focusing knobs and interchangeable lenses of 25 mm to 38 mm are available. Beam-splitters allow viewing the procedure on the video monitor and directly through the endoscope at the same time (Fig. 13-7).

One of the best methods for documenting the hysteroscopic technique to teach, instruct, and review is with a video tape. The tapes are particularly useful for students, nurses, or patients who wish to review the examination. To obtain this documentation, a small, lightweight camera is necessary so the examination can be performed with minimal difficulty. Two types of video cameras are available, the chip and the tube camera. The tube camera has become almost obsolete. Some of these units adapt automatically to the light required depending on the characteristics and the proximity of the hysteroscope to the tissue being observed. Since a potent light source is required, the 300 W xenon lamp is essential.

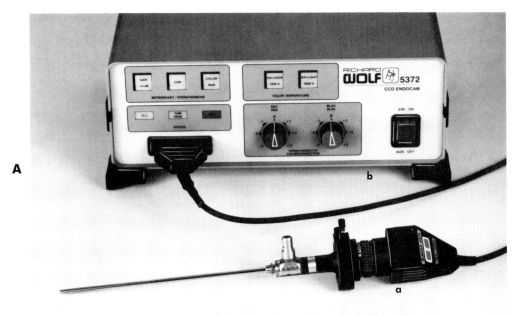

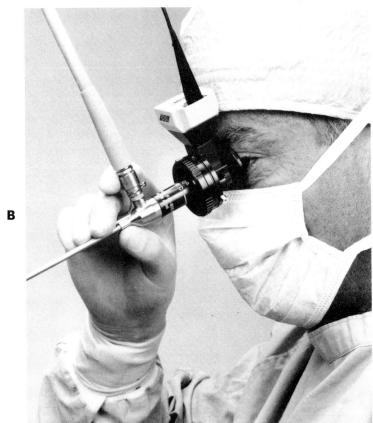

*FIG. 13-7* **A,** Camera head (*a*) weighs 88 g and is attached to hysteroscope and camera controller (*b*). **B,** This chip camera permits direct viewing by surgeon and same image appears on video monitor.

## Monitors and Video Recorders

The picture quality and the system capability of any video equipment depend on the performance of the camera, but an excellent camera and the quality of its image and the reliability of the system cannot be maintained without a monitor and videocassette recorder (VCR) of comparable quality. The operator should be able to connect 2 VCRs (½″ or ¾″) to the monitor. All monitors and VCRs should have hospital-grade plugs and meet or exceed biomedical requirements. Specifications include the size of screen (14″ to 19″), at least 400 lines of resolution, and total remote control. A mobile cart can transport the entire system (Fig. 13-8).

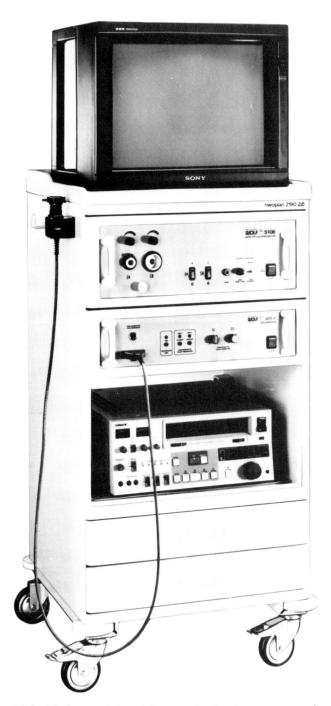

*FIG. 13-8* Special mobile cart obtained to accommodate the monitor, light source, camera head, and controller; video printer can make hard copies.

**Printers**

The video system is enhanced when a high-quality color photograph is electronically produced in seconds (Fig. 13-9). The desired image is captured in digital memory from a television screen or video tape and recorded on film by using a remote foot-control. The image used produces 35 mm slides, negatives for prints, or 3 × 5 Polaroid color prints which can be included in the patient's record.

## CINEMATOGRAPHY

Video recording has replaced 8 mm and 16 mm cinematography. This method has become inappropriate for recording endoscopic procedures because of the complicated process of editing and the cost and weight of the cameras.

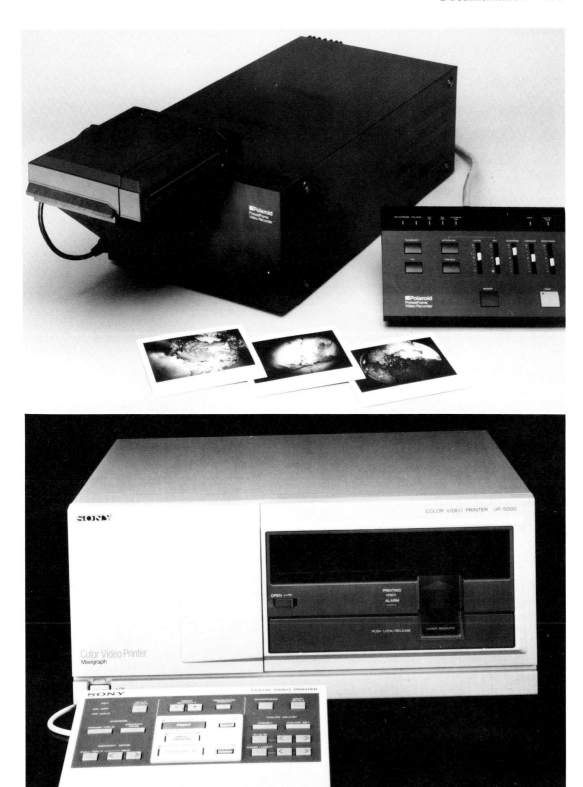

*FIG. 13-9* Video printers produce high-quality 3 × 5 color still pictures (*a,b*).

## TEACHING ATTACHMENTS

The examination can be viewed by several people when teaching attachments are used, and there are several types available (Fig. 13-10). Rigid, straight teaching attachments give the viewer the same picture as the operator and only require an adaptor for the eyepiece. This system does not allow the versatility needed in these situations. Flexible attachments permit perspective that is simultaneous and similar by both observer and surgeon.

Another alternative, the articulated optical arm, maintains good image quality. It is available with 2, 3, and 4 joints depending on the length desired. Despite efforts to prevent loss of light, illumination for the observer is invariably reduced by interfaces; therefore, an integrated attachment is desirable when these teaching devices are used.

## SUMMARY

Endoscopic photography can be enjoyable and enlightening for the surgeon. Take several pictures, carefully note the source of the material, edit seriously, and discard the poor quality images. Only the best films should be retained for demonstration or reproduction purposes.

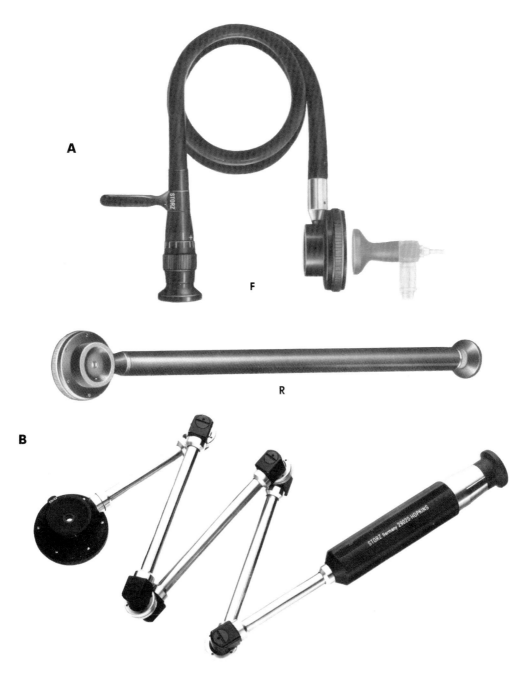

*FIG. 13-10* **A,** Teaching attachments can be rigid (*R*) or flexible (*F*). **B,** Articulated arm can be adjusted so light can be changed from a 50-50 (surgeon-observer) position to a 10-90 position. Photographs can be taken from teaching end of apparatus.

# Index